About the Author

Dr Asrar Rashid
MBChB MRCP MRCPCH DTM&H

Dr Asrar Rashid has been teaching the PLAB for some time and is the main co-author in the series of PLAB books by Medicbyte. He graduated from Scotland and then worked for the President of the Royal College of Paediatrics whilst training as a Paediatrician. He was Successful in the MRCP examination and then went on to be awarded the MRCPCH. His extensive experience in Medicine also includes studying at the Liverpool school of Tropical Medicine and training in anaesthesia. He had a memorable time transporting sick children in New South Wales, Australia and has also had a short stint in Rio De Janeiro, Brazil.

Dr Asrar Rashid is an instructor for the Advanced Paediatric Life Support Group and he enjoys teaching at Undergraduate and Postgraduate level.

Medicbyte

Medicbyte

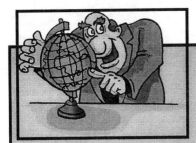

Medicbyte™

Medicbyte™ PLAB Guides!

Are you worried about taking examinations and whether your knowledge is up to scratch? Having problems trying to work out what's important and what to chuck in the litter bin? Do you have to take medical examinations and you haven't much time?
Then the Medicbyte®...... PLAB Guide series is for you!

Medicbyte™ PLAB Best Sellers Guides

.... Medicbyte™ books are written by doctors in plain English.

This PLAB 2 book provides advice specific to the PLAB examination.

A Great Approach to studying for a difficult examination
- PLAB Student

A leading force helping doctors to work in the UK
-Medicpages.com Working in the UK

I found the CDROM which provides access to vital online Videos very helpful indeed
-PLAB 2 Examinee

**Medicbyte®
Global-Books**

| New York | Sydney | Toronto | London |

Medicbyte

1

Medicbyte

OSCE HISTORY EXAMINATION
PLAB 2
Clinical Book

With Interactive CDROM attached!!

By Dr Asrar Rashid

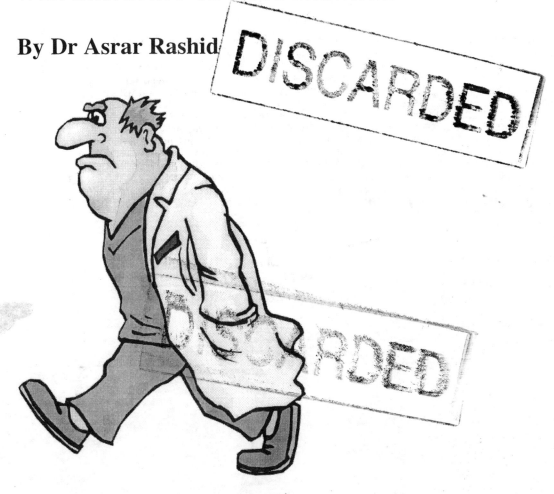

A Book for the UK Medical System
© **Medicbyte 2004**

© Medicbyte 2004   Medicbyte provides **PLAB courses and Videos** for the PLAB examinations
www.medicbyte.com for up to date information on the PLAB & Medicbyte Overseas Centres

Medicbyte

Published by

Medicbyte
55 Leicester Road
Luton
LU4 8SF

Published 2001
Second Edition 2004

Email: plab@medicbyte.com

www.medicbyte.com for details about the PLAB examination

www.medicpages.com for other examination listings and for working in the USA

Copyright © Directbyte 2004

ISBN: 1-904681-00-X

Printed in the United Kingdom

Distributed in the UK by Medicbyte Distributions.

**Medicbyte®
Global-Books**

Medicbyte

Medicbyte

'The biggest secret to passing is to focus on your Patients and <u>not</u> the examiner!

Dr Asrar Rashid
Medicbyte PLAB teacher

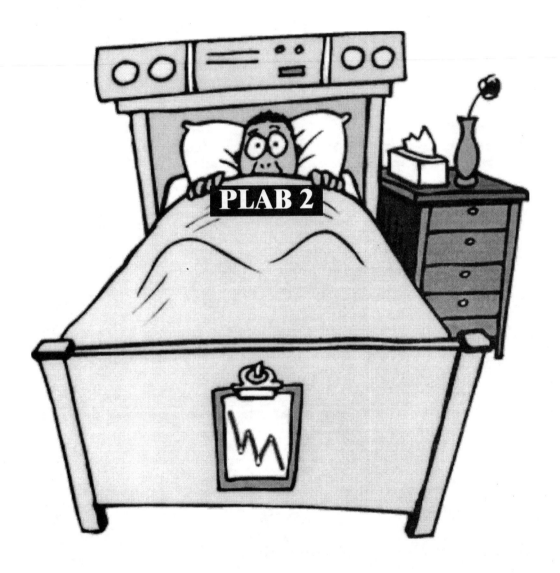

Medicbyte

Foreword

In my experience of teaching the PLAB, doctors who focus on the needs of patients, who have empathy and can reassure; who demonstrate humanity, will be successful in the PLAB and invariably be good clinical practitioners.

This book is for those taking the PLAB part two examination. Medicbyte books for the PLAB have become compulsory reading for doctors preparing for this examination because material is geared to doctors who have never practised in the United Kingdom.

Whatever your background, you must prepare as well as possible. By definition, doctors taking the PLAB part two have worked outside the British medical system and therefore it is imperative that you get used to the way clinical medicine is practised in the United Kingdom. There is no doubt, that like me, you will have learnt something from the PLAB experience that will help you to care for the patients of the future.

Remember that this is the last lap in the marathon to being successful in the PLAB and becoming registered to work in the United Kingdom. The website **www.medicbyte.com** has further important resources for the PLAB 1 and 2 examinations. Attached is a CDROM which provides further interactive information for students using the latest technological advances in e-learning.

This book has not been designed to be a comprehensive text detailing all technique and methodology required for clinical technique but a survival guide for the PLAB.

This text will help you to map out a route to success in the PLAB examination.

I welcome your feedback about the book and wish you all the best. Using the CDROM you can also link into the website and have a look at some online videos and our extensive audio library.

Dr Asrar Rashid
MBChB MRCP MRCPCH DTM&H
Medicbyte PLAB tutor.

Please email me at: plab@medicbyte.com

Medicbyte

Medicbyte

Introduction

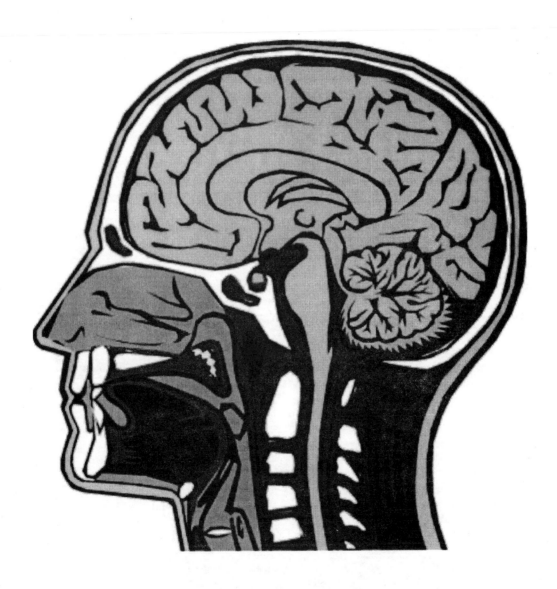

Medicbyte

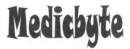
Medicbyte

About the examination- An Introduction

The PLAB test doctors to ensure that they will be able to function as house officers/senior house officers within the UK medical system. Unfortunately the PLAB examination is not a guarantee of a job. This is another hurdle that is addressed briefly in later chapters.

You must learn methodology that is taught throughout the UK medical school system for history taking and clinical examination.

The PLAB 2 consists of a 14 station **O**bjective **S**tructured **C**linical **E**xamination (**OSCE**).

The examination is difficult for overseas doctors having never worked in the United Kingdom. Ideally a clinical attachment should have been undertaken. The PLAB (part 2) examination is designed to test history taking, counselling and practical skills. Marking such an examination is usually very subjective. The objectivity has been introduced through the introduction of the OSCE. The OSCE is used throughout the British clinical curriculum in postgraduate and undergraduate examinations. The OSCE focuses on core skills required to perform as a clinician and therefore applies theory to everyday practice.

If you are the kind of doctor that likes clinical examination and is good at interacting with patients, you will do well. If you aren't then don't worry, read on...

Here are frequent questions asked by examinees:-

How hard is the PLAB 2 examination?

You are not expected to be 'membership standard'. All that is required is that you demonstrate that you can perform to a level expected of a SHO in the United Kingdom. As opposed to other countries the doctors would be thought of as a 'capable SHO' if you demonstrate a good practical working knowledge that would stand you in good stead at any National Health Service Hospital.

What topics does the PLAB 2 cover?

Clinical management topics are included in this examination and only theory that is immidiately applicable to the practical situation will be tested. For example you would be expected to know that taking oral theopyllines is a contraindication to starting intravenous aminoyhilline in asthmatics because of potential toxicity of this drug which has a dangerous toxicity profile.

How is it best to prepare for this examination?

Firstly looks at the way this book is divided into the main areas tested in the OSCE. You should concentrate on each area in turn. More importantly you should get feedback from your friends/ colleagues about what they feel your strengths and weaknesses are. You should then concentrate on these.

Are there real patients involved?

Because the GMC is trying to standardise this examination actors are used that give a standard history and display consistent signs. In some stations manikins will be used, e.g. when you are asked to perform CPR.

How long is required to prepare for the PLAB 2?

This depends on your previous clinical experience and training.

Medicbyte

Medicbyte

'There is no way that anyone can test the depth of your knowledge in 5 Minutes'.

The PLAB 2 is not about knowledge but how you use your skills- communication, interaction- and whether you are sensible, logical and methodological.

About the OSCE examination

1.   14 clinical scenarios and rest stations where there will be no scenarios, each lasts five minutes.

2.   You have one minute to read the instructions before the station begins, outside the station room.

3.   Once inside the OSCE examination room, you stand outside your first station, when the bell rings you can go inside.

4.   There the examiner will make sure you have understood the instructions and you can them begin.

5.   Another bell will ring at 4 and half minutes. Then at five minutes you will have to leave your station.

6.   You then move to your next station.

Just follow the instructions given to you as much as you can at each station.

Each station is broken down for marking purposes into a number of objectives and each objective is weighted. For example if history is only a small part of that station it will not make much of the final percentage of the final mark for that station. Each objective will be given a mark A-E and then the final mark for that objective calculated.

A   Excellent
B   Good
C   Adequate
D   Fail
E   Severe Fail

This is an attempt to apply objectivity to a very subjective clinical situation. However because the examiners are fixed to each station they can best judge how each doctor does against a certain standard.

Medicbyte

Medicbyte

Top Tips

For The PLAB Examination

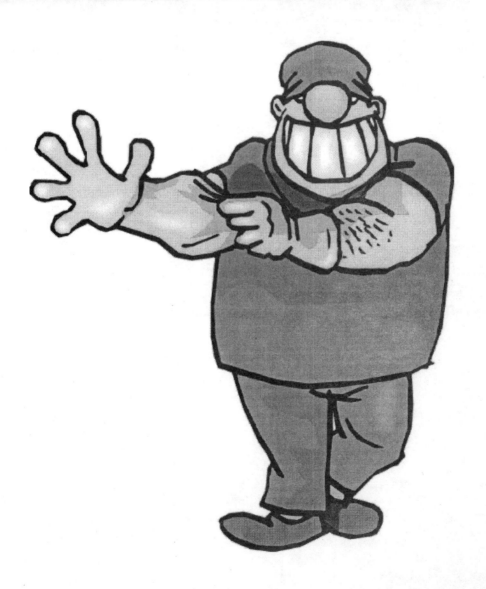

Medicbyte

Medicbyte

Top tips for the PLAB part two

This book by Medicbyte covers important PLAB part two topics.

Important hints for the examination are given below.

This is a really important chapter because these skills are 90% of what is required to be successful.

Practice

Practising scenarios with your colleagues and friends and talking 'medicine' is the best form of preparation. Repetition is the mother of skill.

Think Patient

Remember the examiner is not just after 'a diagnosis' he /she will be looking at your approach to the patient and your courtesy to the patient.

Modelling (a Psychologists technique)

If you have the chance of seeing other doctors at work try to look at what they are doing. What is their approach to the patient? How do they interact? In the 'good' doctors try to model these skills, because modelling will save you much time.

This behavioural technique is often used to develop doctors' skills in a shorter time span. In preparing for the PLAB two preparation think of yourself as the actor who has to 'act' in front of examiners. Practice through role-playing and repetition will make you look polished and experienced on the big day.

Why not watch medical dramas on TV? Learn how the actors interact with colleagues and patients. Don't forget that some of the situations in the PLAB will be of you talking to patents, nurses and senior colleagues. You will be ask to talk directly to patients or role play via a make-up phone.

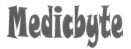

HINTS ON PLEASING THE EXAMINER

If the examiner is pleased, you get more marks. Below are a set of pointers for pleasing the examiner.

Courtesy to patients and family

Ensure you have blinds and curtains around the patient when examining

Ask the patient if he/she feels pain before 'inflicting' pain (remember to look at the patients face if you are about to undertake something that the patient may find painful)

Greet the patient and remember to say goodbye

Help the patient as much as you can- remember they are there of their own free accord and examiners will not tolerate discourtesy.

Be mature in your approach, but not condescending to the patient

If you know the answer put it across in a modest manner without seeming shy, or the other extreme, bullish.

Examination nerves- don't do anything silly!!

So you are on your last stretch, you cannot afford to let nerves take over, you must be yourself on the day. No doctor wishes to be discourteous but under the duress of the examination some actions may appear seem insensitive. Above all, remember that the examiners are in fact human, and they are there to sift out 'dangerous' doctors.

Please…. thank you

You must aim to be polite in the PLAB 2 examination. However; try not to over emphasize this. Remembering your manners can be difficult in the stress associated with the exam!!

Medicbyte

You already know what they will ask!!

The good thing about this examination is that the PLAB 2 is meant to be an objective exercise with candidates scoring points if they undertake certain tasks. It is important that during the preparation for the examination, doctors need to consider the kind of tasks that you will be asked. In clinical medicine there are only a given number of scenarios for 'basic' training, and the candidate would be well advised to be rehearsed in the standard given scenarios that appear commonly in the PLAB. Examples will be given in this book.

Remember the bottom line is that British Hospitals are looking for doctors who will be safe and kind to patients. Reports will be obtained about you in your first 12 months of limited registration once you start work after passing the PLAB examination.

You already know what they will ask!!

The ideal doctor:-

If you were unwell and wanted someone to treat you, I am sure the ideals, given below, would apply.

The doctor must:-

Appearing neat and tidy.

Have a logical approach to questioning that leads to a certain direction.

Remembers the important differential diagnoses.

Can empathize and reassure- picks up non-verbal clues.

Is in control of the situation.

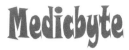

ARRANGING INVESTIGATIONS

At various stations you may be asked to choose investigations either as part of a resuscitation scenario or a counseling scenario.

Medicbyte GOLDEN TIP	When choosing investigations for UK patients you must remember that the UK medical system is a National Health Service and is said to be an ideal model of a health system where patients do not pay at the point of contact.

Consequently it is imperative that you understand that expensive investigations tend not to be first line unless there is a specific diagnostic or therapeutic reason for the investigation.

Medicbyte TOP TIP	Always stick to investigations that you know and not new esoteric techniques that are of research value.

In the USA the story is different where management is sometimes governed by the fear of litigation.

Here are a few examples of important 'investigations'

1. Remembering to do a peak flow measurement on an asthmatic.
2. Remembering to do a blood pressure measurement on a cardiac patient.
3. Remembering to ask for a cross match in a patient about to go to theatre for high-risk surgery (from the blood point of view).
4. Remembering to ask for a blood glucose in a fitting child
5. Remembering to undertake blood cultures in a sepsis scenario
6. Remembering to undertake a rectal core temperature measurement in someone in VF

Medicbyte

Privacy – A Sure Way to Fail!

There are certain scenarios in which the GMC are very strict, please adhere to the points below

1. Intimate Examinations

Medicbyte

Things NOT TO SAY (in the exam and everyday life')

'You are going to die'

'You have end stage cancer'

'This will hurt'

'I think you are lying'

'Please don't waste my time'

Medicbyte

HISTORY TAKING AND COMMUNICATION SKILLS

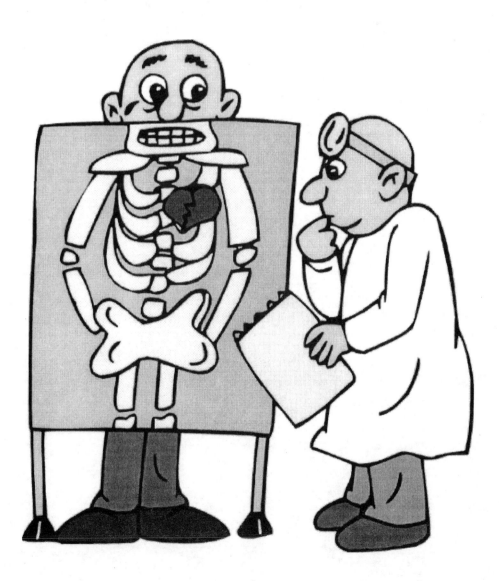

Medicbyte

Medicbyte

This section looks briefly at history taking and communication skills. The concepts in this section will then be practised in the next section.

History Taking and Communication skills

In this, the history and counselling part of the examination you are asked to perform 'role-playing'. This is just like acting and can be unnerving.

However, again, this section of the examination is vital to your function as a doctor in the United Kingdom. Skills can be taught but are often acquired through interactive learning by talking to patients.

For examination preparation you can practice the required skills with your friends and colleagues and more importantly you can see exactly how these are utilised by attending hospitals wards and lectures during your clinical attachment.

At the end of the day the successful clinician must be able to interact with the patient. Filter out unwanted detail and derive a list of differential diagnoses. You will not be expected to list menisci, but you will be expected to have a logical problem solving approach.

In counselling stations you should *always remember your patient*…. What must they be thinking? …. What must he/she be thinking? Putting yourself in the place of your patient will make you empathic and you will the 'see' the important points. The GMC really stress this point and particularly want you to be aware of legal and ethical issues as set out on the GMC publication 'Duties of a Doctor'.

In addition the counselling stations test your true command of language and non-verbal communication.

Aim of this Chapter

In this chapter we will analyse some important scenarios and important points for the examination will be outlined in each. Skills learnt here will also be of value in other aspects of this the part of the examination.

Remember, practice, practice, and practice!

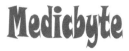

HISTORY TAKING

Remember in the history remember the following points:-

- Concentrate on those areas that are specific to the complaint or question being posed by the examiner otherwise you will not score highly.
- How you put the questions and how you respond to the patient will be scrutinised.
- You will find that a number of skills you gain for the counselling station can also be used effectively in history taking.
- **You only have 5 minutes per station** so your questioning should be precise and to the point.
- Once the main point has been addressed you should also consider other points that may be important such as a past medical history.

A full history would normally take the format of

1. Presenting complaint
2. History of presenting complaint
3. Past medical history
4. Drug history
5. Social history
6. Systematic enquiry.

Obviously you will not have time to take a complete history, which normally takes 30 minutes. Instead you must formulate a plan for the likely topics that will come up in the examination.

ORDER THE MEDICBYTE EXAMINATION VIDEOS ONLINE NOW!! YOU CAN DO THIS FROM THE WEBSITE AT WWW.MEDICBYTE.COM

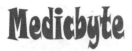

A FOCUSED HISTORY IS THE KEY

STEPS:

1.Read the question.

2.Decide which system is involved

3.Think of questions focusing on the differential diagnosis.

4.Formulate a differential diagnosis and a management plan.

"I found, practicing different scenarios with my friends was helpful in getting me to
to focus on various clinical problems."

Asima Kishur

Medicbyte TOP TIP	When you are under the pressure of the examination if you can achieve points 1 to 3 before you enter into the station then you will be in a strong position

IMPORTANT POINT: TAILOR YOUR HISTORY TO THE PATEINT

Ok, here is an exercise...

Imagine you are asked to talk to a patient about changing Life Style post myocardial infarction, what would you ask? Take a minute to jot down some important questions.

Some questions are extremely important. For example if you forget to ask a patient who has recently had a Myocardial Infarction about smoking then you will lose points. From now until the examination think about these important scenarios.

REMEMBER THE PATIENT

When asking the patient questions you must really focus on the patient. Here are helpful tips from past candidates:-

1. The stations in the examination are quite standard. However the PLAB 2 isn't like an examination where if you know the answer beforehand it will help in getting the best marks.
2. Learn the type of questions you must ask for each of the main conditions so that on the day it seems that you have been practicing medicine all your life.
3. In your questions be sensitive to your patient. If you patient says that he/she has a worry you must allay this worry.
4. The patient is the main person in all this and you should be putting yourself in his/her place. What are his feelings; why is he/she feeling sad? What are the important issues for the patient?
5. It's hard to forget you are being examined; however the doctor that can act the best in this nervy environment will breeze through the examination.

You only have one minute to organise your thoughts and you will do well to practice beforehand.

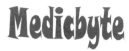

COMMUNICATION- Core skills

Although communication will be tested throughout the OSCE through
your interaction with the actors there are specific situations in which the skill is tested.

Below are examples of the type of skills you will need:-

You should be able to talk to patients about, diagnoses and investigations
Discuss understanding
Talk to relatives
Break bad news
Dealing with angry individuals
Talk about lifestyle changes in relation to important public health issues such as smoking.
You may have to check your patients understanding of important issues
Discuss important blood tests
Talk to 'difficult' patients

Medicbyte

Non-verbal communication techniques

Communication is a complex discipline, which is not only achieved by use of human language but also through non-verbal techniques.

- *Mirroring*

This is when you copy your examiner or patient posture and mood. Psychologists say that the correct application of this will allow you to develop a positive relationship with your examiner or patient quickly.

All you do is mirror the stance and posture of the opposite person. This should be done subtly and not obviously. Mirroring does not have to be exact. Clearly this tool requires a lot of work. From now on watch it being used in everyday life and see if you can adopt it to your advantage.

- *Sitting and Seating arrangements*

Seating and the way you sit is often neglected when looking at the patient doctor interaction. It is very important to have a good balance between being distant and overbearing as opposed to being close and too invading the patient's space.

In the PLAB examination you will be herded from place to place so that you and all the other candidates stay close to time. The seating will probably be pre planned therefore be able to assume a seating stance that is comfortable for you at each station. Your seating posture is so important for you to be able to provide a comfortable persona and impress the examiner.

- *Hands*

Different cultural groups use their hands differently and you should be aware of your hands in the consultation and also when you present anything in front of the examiner. As a rule hands should be used seldom in the interaction with the patient and when presenting to the examiners.

- *Eyes*

Again this is cultural variation as to the level of application of eye contact. On the whole eye contact should be maintained with the patient or examiner most of the time. Although this should not be overdone as to seem aggressive and artificial. Over the next few weeks watch doctors and people talking and notice all the aspects of the interaction process.

Medicbyte

Important verbal techniques

- *Saying 'yes,....I see....'*

This is to help encourage the patient to talk about the problem.

In the PLAB you will probably have to lead the patient down the desired route to score effectively. In real life you will get patients whom may not be to the point and in fact may need a lot of prompting to stay on track.

- *'That is interesting....but coming back to the point about ...'*

Some patients forget about the point asked and may veer off at a tangent. The above phrase will help them focus on the point at hand.

- *'You were telling me about........'*

This helps the patient to focus on a particular point.

It is unlikely that the patients that are used in the examination will deliberately go off at a tangent, but how quickly you get answers to the problem at hand will depend on your precise question asking ability.

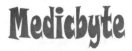

Presenting your findings to the examiner

The presentation of your findings is important, as this will test your ability to pass on valuable information.

You must be able to demonstrate the following: -

- You can organise facts (mentioning the important facts first and the not so important last)
- You can communicate effectively with your peers
- That you do not make up facts
- That you have conviction in yourself, but at the same time, you are not arrogant- there is a perception that doctors should always be prepared to learn from their mistakes and the more arrogant you are the more unlikely you are open to correction.

Medicbyte Tips for Presenting to the examiners

- *Look at the examiner-* eye contact or near eye contact is practised in the United Kingdom. When you are talking to the examiner make sure that

- *Rationalise the information you are about to present-* know what you need to tell the examiner and where it will lead you. If you know that a certain diagnosis is likely ensure that your findings conform to this; but do not make up findings that do not exist.

- *Don't expect feedback.* In real life when you talk to your peers you expect a bit of head nodding or noises of disagreement. The examiners will try not to give you any feedback and most will appear very plain faced and none-helpful. DON'T BE disorientated by this- this is an exam and is not real life!

The best way to practise this before your examination is to talk to yourself and others about 'made up' findings. Talking to the mirror is also a good way of practising presentation. The more you the more likely your actions and words will appear second nature on the big day!

Medicbyte

Medicbyte

History taking and Communication

Worked Examples by Medicbyte

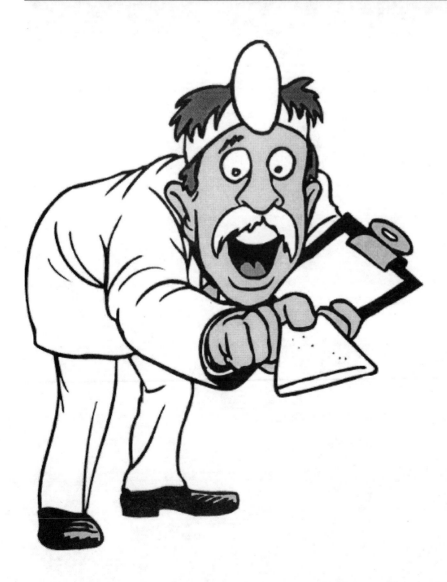

Medicbyte

Medicbyte

In this section we will ask you to go through some worked examples.

Take one minute as you read each example to scribble down what YOU will ask the patient in the actual examination.......

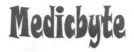

HISTORY AND COMMUNICATION 1

Childhood cough- instructions to candidates

This station tests your ability to come to a diagnosis

- *Mrs Jameson has brought her five year old to your GP surgery with a night time cough*
- *Ask the relevant questions to elucidate the diagnosis*

This station lasts five minutes

Now list the questions YOU will ask below:-

1..
....
2..
....
3..
....
4..
....
5..
....
6..
....
7..
....
8..
....
9..
....
10..
....

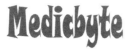

WHAT THE EXAMINER IS LOOKING FOR:-

CONSTRUCT

The candidate demonstrates the ability to take a history and reach a diagnosis in an effective way in a case of nocturnal childhood cough

OBJECTIVES

1. Communication
   Establishes rapport
   Listens attentively
   Uses appropriate questioning strategies

2. Elicits adequate presenting complaint
   Elicits a history of asthma
   Checks chronicity
   Checks risk factors

3. Other history
   Takes a good social history
   Checks family history

4. Diagnosis
   Suggests a diagnosis

Learning Points

Asthma is an important and common clinical condition for it to appear in the examination in many guises from diagnosis through to acute and chronic treatment.

The scenario where you are asked to reassure a parent or talk to a parent appears in many guises in the PLAB and in real life.

You should be able to communicate effectively and address the main parental concerns if you are to score well. Other scenarios that may occur include the child with a petechial rash or the child with diarrhea (I am worried he is dehydrated doctor).

Know about   Asthma Risk factors
Therapeutic aspects include step up and step down therapy
Medical devices for asthmatics
Emergency treatment and diagnosis

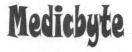

HISTORY AND COMMUNICATION 2

Tiredness and polyuria-instructions to candidates

This station tests your ability to come to a diagnosis

- *28 year old Jim,has been feeling tired for the last 3 weeks*
- *He also has been having increased frequency of micturition*

This station lasts for five minutes

Now list the questions YOU will ask below:-

1..
....
2..
....
3..
....
4..
....
5..
....
6..
....
7..
....
8..
....
9..
....
10..
....

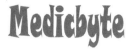

WHAT THE EXAMINER IS LOOKING FOR:

CONSTRUCT

Your ability to ask appropriate questions to reach the correct diagnosis.

OBJECTIVES

1. Communication
   Brief introduction
   Establish rapport
2. Listen to the presenting complaints carefully
   Ask relavant question
3. The duration of symptoms
   The frequency of micturition
   History of thirst
   Any increase in appetite
   Loss of weight
4. Family history of diabetes
   Past medical and surgical history
5. Diagnosis
   Suggest a diagnosis.

Learning points

The symptoms suggest diabetes, typically, type I
The patient being young, presenting with polyuria, polydypsia and polyphagia.
Complaining of fatigue.
There may be a family history,
The investigations are measuring the blood sugar,
Glucose tolerance test
Treatment includes diet care and insulin,
Oral hypoglycemics are not used in type I diabetes patients

There are only a few common causes of polyuria- the most important being diabetes Mellitus and Urinary Tract infections.

> **'Beware the 7 year old with tiredness'**
> **- ask about   polyuria and polydipsia**

Medicbyte

COMPLICATIONS OF DIABETES

ACUTE:

Hypoglycemic episode

Ketoacidotic emergency

Both conditions can lead to unconsciousness and coma.

OTHER COMPLICATIONS:

1. Vascular complications

2. Increased susceptibility to infection

3. Diabetic neuropathy

4. Diabetic nephropathy

5. Diabetic retinopathy

6. Diabetic foot   (due to infection, loss of sensation and vascular effects)

Diabetes is one of the classic conditions in the examination that can present in several different ways and has a number of different management facets.

Medicbyte

DIFFERENTIATING BETWEEN HYPOGLYCEMIC COMA & KETOACIDOTIC COMA

HYPOGLYCEMIC COMA

KETOACIDOTIC COMA

HISTORY:

Excessive insulin intake
Decreased food intake
Unusual exercise

Reduced amount of insulin,
h/o overeating, under activity
complaint of other
Complications
The patient 's condition
gradually deteriorates

COMMON SYMPTOMS:

Sweating
Hunger, anxiety
Confusion
Drowsiness
Nausea
Headache
Tiredness
Irritability

Nausea, vomiting,
intense thirst
It may be associated with
Abdominal pain
Increased urine output

EXAMINATION:

Skin and tongue are moist
The pulse is full
Systolic blood pressure may be
Normal
Breathing maybe normal or shallow
Tendon reflexes are brisk

Dry skin and tongue
Pulse is weak
BP is low
Patient maybe gasping for air
Reflexes are diminished

INVESTIGATIONS:

URINE

No ketonuria
No Glycosuria

ketonuria
and glycosuria
Usually present

BLOOD

Hypoglycaemia
Plasma bicarbonate level
Maybe normal

Hyperglycaemia
reduced plasma
bicarbonate

Medicbyte

FOLLOW-UP OF DIABETIC PATIENTS

AT ROUTINE CHECKUPS:

Ask the patient to keep a record of hypoglycaemic episodes experienced.

Check Peripheral pulses

Check Blood pressure

Check Record routine body weight

Urine analysis: Ketones
                      Albumin(for kidney function)
                      Glucose
                      Evidence of UTI

Blood: Glucose

                Glycosylated haemoglobin

Ocular examination

Ophthalmoscopy

Neurological exam:
                Sensation in the limbs
                Motor function
                Reflexes

Examine feet for any evidence of diabetic foot

- Ulceration,
- Gangrene,
- Infection

Medicbyte

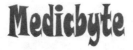

HISTORY AND COMMUNICATION 3

Dealing with anxiety surrounding the diagnosis of meningitis-instructions to the candidates

This station tests your ability to reassure

- *A teacher phones you on the ward. You have just admitted a 9-year old boy with meningitis*
- *Niesseria Meningitides has been isolated from the blood cultures*

Allay the teachers concerns about the risks to other children by talking to her

This station lasts five minutes.

Now list the questions YOU will ask below:-

1...
....
2...
....
3...
....
4...
....
5...
....
6...
....
7...
....
8...
....
9...
....
10...
....

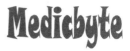

WHAT THE EXAMINER IS LOOKING FOR:-

CONSTRUCT

You should be able to listen to the teacher and allay her fears about the risk to other children at school.

OBJECTIVES

1. Communication
   Listen carefully
   Ask appropriate questions according to her concerns.
2. Give the teacher a brief description of early symptoms and that any child showing such
   Symptoms be taken to a doctor as soon as possible.
3. Tell her that Public Health doctors will be contacting the school.
   Close contacts of the child with the infection will be given 'medicine' by the Public health doctors.
   It will be up to the public health doctors to decide who needs treating.
   Vaccination for unimmunised children will also be arranged by the public health doctors

Important questions that the teacher ask may include:

1. What is meningitis?
2. How can it be prevented?
3. Whom should I contact?

Learning points

Usually the close contacts of the index case of meningitis will be treated. The responsibly for this is usually via Public Health. The doctor on call admitting the patient should phone the public health team. Remember that there are many causes of meningitis, but it is the bacterial form (N meningitides), which requires prophylaxis in contacts. Please refer to the PLAB 1 books regarding the topic of prophylaxis.

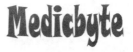

HISTORY AND COMMUNICATION 4

Difficulty in micturition- instructions to candidates

This station tests your ability to come to a diagnosis

- *Mr Jones been referred to the general surgical clinic because of a three week history of difficulty in micturition.*
- *Ask the relevant questions to elucidate the diagnosis*

This station lasts five minutes

Now list the questions YOU will ask below:-

1..
....

2..
....

3..
....

4..
....

5..
....

6..
....

7..
....

8..
....

9..
....

10..
....

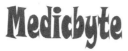

WHAT THE EXAMINER IS LOOKING FOR:-

CONSTRUCT

You should be able to ask appropriate questions in order to make the right diagnosis.

OBJECTIVES

1. Communication
   Brief introduction
2. Listen to the presenting complaints
   Elicit comprehensive history
   Ask about frequency
   The stream of urine
   Any dribbling after passing urine
   Any pain or burning
3. briefly ask other history
   as family history and past medical and surgical history
4. Diagnosis
   Suggest a diagnosis

Learning Points

The history of difficult micturition in an aged man associated with increased frequency,
poor stream and dribbling of urine typically suggests prostatic enlargement that is benign prostatic
hyperplasia.The condition has to be differentiated from prostatic carcinoma,in which the history will
suggest weight loss,general weakness and any metastaic symptoms.Clinical examination is also very
important in differentiating the two conditions.The treatment for BPH is surgical,TURP(transurethral
resection of the prostate)being the most popular technique.

Medicbyte

CAUSES VARIOUS URINARY CONDITIONS

DIFFICULTY IN PASSING URINE

(CAN LEAD TO RETENTION IF OBSTRUCTION IN THE URINARY PASSAGE IS COMPLETE)

Obstruction in the lumen :

- Congenital anomalies of the urinary system(rare)

- Foreign bodies stones

- Tumours Etc.

In the wall:

- Strictures

- Prostate enlargement

- Tumour

- Trauma/rupture

Outside:

- Faecal impaction

- Paraphimosis (in males)

- Pregnancy

- Fibroids

- Ovarian cyst (in females)

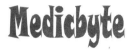

Other causes:

- In the post-operative period

- Spinal cord injuries/

- Diseases

- Drugs (anticholinergics, anti-histamines, muscle relaxants etc)

- Other disease of the urinary system.

Medicbyte

PAINFUL MICTURITION:

- Infection

- Rupture

- Bladder carcinoma

- Other conditions of the urethra

FREQUENCY:

- Renal tuberculosis

- Vesical calculous

- Prostatic enlargement

- Benign

- Malignant

- Urethral narrowing (due to strictures)

Medicbyte

HAEMATURIA

THIS CAN BE CLASSIFIED ACCORDING TO DIFFERENT SITES:

KIDNEY

- Tumours   Wilm's
                     Transitional cell ca

- Glomerulonephritis

- Tuberculosis

- Injury

- Infarct

URETER

- Tumor

- Stone

BLADDER

- Cystitis

- Shistosomiasis

- Tumour

- Stones

URETHRA:

- Rupture

- Stone

- Prostate(benign/malignant)

GENERAL CAUSES OF HAEMATURIA

- Haemophilia

- Malaria

- Scurvy

- Purpura

- Anticoagulants

TYPICAL SYMPTOMS OF PROSTATISM

- Frequency

- Urgency

- Difficulty in passing urine

- Poor stream

- Terminal dribbling

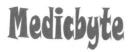

HISTORY AND COMMUNICATION 5

Contraceptive advice- instructions to candidates

This station tests your ability to counsel patients about contraceptive advice

- *Miss Ferdinand, a 25-year-old lady, comes to you for advice on contraception*
- *Give the relevant advice*

This station lasts five minutes

Now list the questions YOU will ask below:-

1..
....
2..
....
3..
....
4..
....
5..
....
6..
....
7..
....
8..
....
9..
....
10..
....

Medicbyte

WHAT THE EXAMINER IS LOOKING FOR:-

CONSTRUCT

You should be able to communicate properly with the lady, advising her :
the most suitable method and allying her fears about complications.

OBJECTIVES

1. Communication
   Establish rapport
   Tell her it is better to discuss this in the presence of her partner.

2. Take brief history
   Ask about any specific reasons
   Her general health

3. Explain that there are various methods of contraception
   The most commonly used are, the barrier method and the oral contraceptives.
   The method used also depends on the partners.

Important questions that may be asked by the lady:

1. what method would be the most suitable for me?
2. what are the side effects of the oral contraceptives?
3. will there be any problems in conceiving afterwards?
4. what is the link between cancer and contraception?

Learning points

History of hypertension,
Irregular menstruation,
Headaches,migraine
History of hyperlipidemia or CVA in the family.

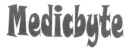
Medicbyte

RISK FACTORS AND CHIEF SYMPTOMS FOR VARIOUS GYNAECOLOGICAL CONDITIONS

Knowing these helps in taking an effective history...

ENDOMETRIOSIS:

RISK FACTORS:

Low parity

Endometriosis is closely associated with primary infertility and is also found to be more common In women with low parity as compared with multiparous women

-Note-
Pregnancy protects against endometriosis as it suppresses ovarian activity

Genetic predisposition

Age group mostly affected (30-40 yrs)

Racial background may have an influence

SYMPTOMS:

- Dysmenorrhia

- Dysparunia

- Abdominal pain ---Intensity depends on acute or chronic condition.

- Menorrhagia

- Infertility

Medicbyte

CERVICAL CARCINOMA:

RISK FACTORS:

- Multiple sexual partners.

- Age at first intercourse

- More common in multipara, indirectly related to low age at first pregnancy thus intercourse.

- Race and religion may have influence

- Smoking has been found to be an associated risk factor

- Viral basis: Human papilloma virus (HPV) has been found to be involved.

SYMPTOMS:

- Irregular vaginal bleeding:

- Inter menstrual,

- Post coital

- Post menopausal

- Pain and discharge are usually associated with complications.

Medicbyte

UTERINE MYOMAS

RISK FACTORS:

- Increased production of oestrogens

- As they occur during childbearing age and regress after menopause

- Common in nulliparous/low parity women

- Racial and genetic factors may be involved

SYMPTOMS:

- Menorrhagia is the main symptom

- Irregular bleeding and Pain is associated with complicated cases

- The patient may complain of a feeling of mass in the lower abdomen

- Pressure symptoms may affect:

    Urinary passage

    GIT

    Lower limb veins (leading to distension and varicosities)

Medicbyte

ENDOMETRIAL CARCINOMA

RISK FACTORS:

- It is a disease of old age.

- Highest incidence after 60 years of age.

- Low parity is a causative factor

- Late menopause

- Overweight women are more susceptible

- Oestrogen overactivity leading to hyperplastic endometrium, predisposes to carcinoma.

- Often associated with myomas

- And senile endometritis

SYMPTOMS:

- Irregular vaginal bleeding

- Pain and

- Discharge

- Are late symptoms.

- Metastatic symptoms due to local and distant spread

Medicbyte

OVARIAN TUMOURS

RISK FACTORS:

- Environmental influence

- Exposure to:

- Chemicals

- Radiation

- Prolonged reproductive period

- Dietary influence

- Genetic effects

SYMPTOMS:

- Abdominal mass/discomfort

- GI and

- Urinary disturbance

- Hormonal effects

- Due to abnormal hormone production e.g masculinization

- Symptoms of malignancy

- Ill health

- Weight loss

- Local and distant metastases

Medicbyte

HYDATIDIFORM MOLE

RISK FACTORS:

- Advanced maternal age

- Women with high parity

- Environmental factors

- Adverse socio-economic conditions

- Previous molar pregnancy

SYMPTOMS:

- Symptoms are those of early pregnancy i.e amenorrhea, but vomiting may be severe leading to

- Hyperemesis gravidarum

- Vaginal bleeding or

- Brownish discharge

- No foetal movement is felt by the mother

Medicbyte

PELVIC INFLAMMATORY DISEASE:

RISK FACTORS:

Ill health/anaemia

Poor living conditions

Multiparity

Repeated births under poor conditions

Difficult or prolonged labour

No use of aseptic techniques

Criminal abortions

Tuberculosis

SYMPTOMS:

- GENERAL:

    Pain

    Fever

    Ill health

- SPECIFIC

    Dysmenorrhia

    Dysparunia

    Infertility(specially genital tuberculosis)

    Menstrual disorders

    Vaginal discharge

Medicbyte

ECTOPIC PREGNANCY

RISK FACTORS:

- Congenitally malformed fallopian tubes

- Pelvic inflammatory disease

- Tuberculous salpingitis

- Intrauterine contraceptive device

- Pelvic tumours

SYMPTOMS:

- Short period of amenorrhea (7-14days)

- Pain

- Usually severe associated with fainting

- Nausea and vomiting

- Vaginal bleeding following pain

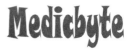

DIFFERENCE BETWEEN

PELVIC INFLAMMATORY DISEASE	**ENDOMETRIOSIS**

These conditions present with common symptoms like:

Dysmenorrhea

Dysparunia

Infertility

The differences are:

PELVIC INFLAMMATORY DISEASE	ENDOMETRIOSIS
The pain in dysmenorrhea is maximum Before the period right up to the onset And is relieved with onset of periods.	The pain gets worse during menstruation going right to the end.
History of abortion/difficult labour May be found.	Not necessarily
Fallopian tubes are blocked, Especially in salpingo-ophoritis.	Usually patent
No response	Respond to hormonal therapy

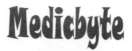

HISTORY AND COMMUNICATION 6

A case of suicide risk- instructions to candidates

This station tests your ability to deal with suicidal patients

- *Speak to Jane, 25 your lady who has tried commit suicide this morning.*
- *A paracetamol container was found by her bedside, empty.*

This station lasts five minutes

Now list the questions YOU will ask below:-

1...
....
2...
....
3...
....
4...
....
5...
....
6...
....
7...
....
8...
....
9...
....
10...
....

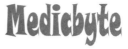

WHAT THE EXAMINER IS LOOKING FOR:-

CONSTRUCT:

Your ability to assess the seriousness of the intent, the reasons behind the attempt and whether she is likely to try again.

OBJECTIVES:

1. Communication
   Make the patient feel comfortable
   Listen to her carefully
2. Firstly you have to ascertain the seriousness of the suicide intent.
   For example if you found written note, saying 'goodbye', this is much more worrying.
   Ask her the reason of this suicide attempt and if she really wanted to die
   Does she intend to repeat this in future
3. The patient needs attention, a lot of reassurance and support
4. If the patient has to be admitted to the hospital and refuses to stay then the mental health officer should be contacted.
5. On admission the nursing staff should be told of the seriousness of suicide risk so that appropriate staff may be assigned to take care of the lady

Learning points:

Patient's mental state,
Severity of the attempt and the intention behind.
Any future plans.

Important questions to ask the patient:

Why did you do this?
Did you want to die?
Do you intend to try again?

The bottom line is this you have to ascertain the level of suicide intent. In clinical practice this judgment and management is left to the on call psychiatrist.

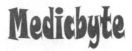

HISTORY AND COMMUNICATION 7

A case of abdominal pain- instructions to candidates

This station tests your ability to

- *Speak to Madelin,. A 25 year old lady with abdominal pain.*
- *Ask her questions that will lead you to a differential diagnosis.*

This station lasts five minutes.

Now list the questions YOU will ask below:-

1...
....
2...
....
3...
....
4...
....
5...
....
6...
....
7...
....
8...
....
9...
....
10...
....

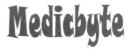

WHAT THE EXAMINER IS LOOKING FOR:-

CONSTRUCT

A short comprehensive history leading to the possible diagnosis.

OBJECTIVES

1. Communication
   brief introduction.
2. Ask about the site of pain
   the severity
   duration
   aggravating and relieving factors
   associated symptoms
   any previous episodes
3. other history
   sexual history
   Past medical and surgical history.

Learning points:

- Remember all the possible differential diagnoses
- Rule out the gynaecological conditions
- The abdominal examination findings are very important in this case
- You may be asked about necessary investigations.

  Investigations depends upon the diagnosis
  Baseline investigations include
  Ultra sound
  X-ray

Medicbyte

ABDOMINAL PAIN:

CAUSES AND IMPORTANT FINDINGS IN HISTORY:

PURELY ABDOMINAL CONDITIONS:

PEPTIC ULCER:

It may present with varying degrees of pain in the abdomen. It depends on the severity and condition of the ulcer,
Severe acute pain may occur in perforated ulcer leading to peritonitis and shock.

DIFFERENT PRESENTATIONS:

GASTRIC ULCER:

Epigastric pain

Usually starts immediately or up to 2 hours after food intake

Aggravated by eating

Relieved by vomiting

Haematemesis may be present

DUODENAL ULCER:

Epigastric pain

Starts usually after 2 years of taking food

Aggravates by missing a meal, stress.

Relieved by eating

RISK FACTORS:

Factors that aggravate the condition are:

Smoking

Alcohol

NSAIDs

Steroids

Excessive tea and coffee intake

Stress and anxiety

Medicbyte

PERFORATED PEPTIC ULCER:

It is an emergency,

The patient presents with severe abdominal pain,

Weakness, pallor faintness

May go into shock if peritonitis ensues.

PANCREATITIS:

ACUTE:

The patient may present with:

Epigastric pain

Radiating to back

Nausea and vomiting

In severe advanced cases hypocalcaemic tetany may develop causing muscular twitching

CHRONIC:

Pain is less severe than acute condition

Anorexia vomiting

Weight loss

Fat indigestion

Symptoms of diabetes may develop as a late feature

CHOLECYSTITIS:

ACUTE:

Pain in hypochondrium

Aggravated by movement

Relieved by analgesics

Nausea vomiting

Fever

Medicbyte

CHRONIC:

Pain radiating to shoulder blade

Duration is usually less than 12 hours

Aggravated by fatty food

Nausea vomiting

Flatulent dyspepsia

APPENDICITIS:

Pain starts in the umbilical region.

Shifting to the right iliac fossa

Anorexia nausea vomiting

Fever

The site of pain is tender, if pressed

INTESTINAL OBSTRUCTION:

Abdominal pain,

Distension

Constipation

Vomiting

Are the features typical?

Other causes in the abdomen:

Acute mesenteric lymphadenitis

Regional ileitis

Meckel's diverticulitis(may be confused with appendicitis)

Carcinoma of the caecum

Medicbyte

GYNAECOLOGICAL CONDITIONS:

Ectopic pregnancy

Ruptured ovarian cyst

Salpingitis

Important points in history:

> History of short ammenorhea(for ectopic pregnancy)
>
> Menstrual irregularities
>
> Previous gynaecological/obstetric history

OTHER CONDITIONS:

RENAL:

Some renal conditions can present with abdominal pain;

Ureteric colic

Acute pyelonephritis

ENDOCRINAL:

Diabetic crisis

BLOOD DISORDERS:

Henoch Shonlein purpura

Porphyria

Medicbyte

DIFFERENTIAL DIAGNOSIS OF BREATHLESSNESS:

CARDIAC FAILURE:

Starts as exertional dyspnoea

Accompanied by pulmonary oedema

Paroxysmal nocturnal dyspnoea

Orthopnea

RESPIRATORY:

Asthma

COPD h/o smoking, cough expectoration

Pneumonia history of fever, resp infection

Pulmonary neoplasms

Airway obstruction

GENERAL:

Psychogenic

Severe anaemia

Inhalation of poisonous gas

Medicbyte

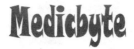

HISTORY AND COMMUNICATION 8

Using a metered dose inhaler- instructions to candidates

This station tests your ability to explain to patients on how to use common devices

- *Speak to Jim, a 8 year old boy is about to begin ventolin via a MDI and a spacer device.*
- *Explain to him how to use the device*

This station lasts five minutes.

Now list the questions YOU will ask below:-

1..
....
2..
....
3..
....
4..
....
5..
....
6..
....
7..
....
8..
....
9..
....
10..
....

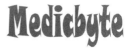

WHAT THE EXAMINER IS LOOKING FOR:-

CONSTRUCT
    Know how to counsel someone about the use of a Metered dose inhaler

OBJECTIVES
1. Communication
   Brief introduction- why it is important and how it works
2. Check to ensure that there is enough drug in the inhaler and then shake the container
3. How to hold the inhaler
4. Synchronising breathing with inhalation of the aerosol
5. How to keep the inhaler clean

Teaching points for MDI administration by patients

MDI ISSUES
    shaking canister
    Priming new or infrequently used inhaler
    Removal of cap before treatment
    Holding the canister correctly
    Assessing when the canister is empty

HOLDING CHAMBER ISSUES
    Preparation of the device (take off cap, attach inhaler)
    Actuation into the chamber
    Priming/Cleaning issues
    Immediate inhalation after loading device

PATIENT ISSUES
    Breathing pattern (inspiratory flow, breath-hold)
    Time between actuation
    Use only as prescribed

Important notes for exam day:

- Ensure the canister is not empty
- Ensure that the patient is breathing at the correct time and in synchrony with MDI activation
- Remember that some patients may have difficulty despite your efforts and may instead need to use a different type of inhaler
- Children and the elderly should be encouraged to use the spacer device when using a MDI system.

The spacer is like a large plastic bottle that can be attached to the MDI. The patient breathes in and out of the spacer when the drug is squirted into it. Different sizes and types of spacers are available

Just remember Ventolin goes with a Volumatic (type of spacer device) as does Becotide (inhaled steroid).

In normal clinical practice in the UK, patients are asked to attend their GP clinic Asthma clinics where technique can be assessed and corrected regularly.

Please note
i. A metered dose inhaler is a common method of drug delivery however other methods are available.
ii. New MDI's are being introduced that are ecologically friendly, these do not contain CFC's and therefore are much lighter and it can sometimes be difficult to assess just how much drug is left.

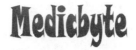

HISTORY AND COMMUNICATION 9

Abnormal pap smear-Instructions to candidates

This station tests your ability to counsel the patient about her report

- *Janet is 36 years old and has an abnormal smear test.(PAP SMEAR)*
- *Counsel her and explain what she has to do about it.*

This station lasts for five minutes.

Now list the questions YOU will ask below:-

1..
....
2..
....
3..
....
4..
....
5..
....
6..
....
7..
....
8..
....
9..
....
10..
....

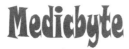

WHAT THE EXAMINER ISLOOKING FOR:-

CONSTRUCT
> Tell her what the abnormal test means and that follow up would be necessary

OBJECTIVES
1. Communication
   brief introduction

2. You've received the report
   tell her that the positive report means,
   there are abnormal cells in the cervix,
   which means there is a high risk of developing cancer

3. She will have to visit her doctor regularly so that the test can be repeated
   Even if it starts getting worse, it would be better to start the treatment as early as possible

Learning points

Risk factors for Cervical cancer

- Women with multiple sexual
- Early commencement of intercourse.
- The Human papilloma virus(HPV) is associated

The prognosis depends on the stage of the disease.

- The earliest stage is cervical intraepithelial neoplasia (CIN) in which the dysplastic changes are confined to the epithelium.
- Further stages I,II,III,IV(all further divided into a, b, c) depend on the involvement of deeper tissues as well as distant metastasis.

Exam Hint	Learn the risk factors for the major conditions so that you can counsel patients about lifestyle changes

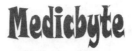

HISTORY AND COMMUNICATION 10

PR bleeding in an old man-Instructions to candidates

This station tests your ability to take a short history to elicit a diagnosis
- *Bill a 65-year old man presents with bleeding PR, take an appropriate history.*
- *Ask appropriate questions to reach a diagnosis*

This station lasts five minutes.

Now list the questions YOU will ask below:-

1...
....
2...
....
3...
....
4...
....
5...
....
6...
....
7...
....
8...
....
9...
....
10...
....

Medicbyte

WHAT THE EXAMINER IS LOOKING FOR:-

CONSTRUCT
Take a brief, comprehensive history comprising of relevant questions.

OBJECTIVES

1. Communication
   establish rapport
2. history should include
   the duration,
   amount of blood,
   colour,
   associated pain,
   relation with defaecation and its effect on it,
   mixed with mucous or faeces,
   any urinary symptoms
3. briefly ask,
   past medical and surgical history
   treatment history(if any)

Learning points

- Bleeding PR can be due to a number of causes, mostly in the lower GIT
- Presence or absence of pain is important- haemorrhoidal bleeding is painless unless infected or complicated
- If Carcinoma of colon and rectum is the cause, bleeding may be painful
- Blood mixed with mucous can occur in inflammatory bowel diseases.
- Other differentials include Angiodysplasia,
    Anal fissure (very painful)
    Rarely it is due to a specific bleeding disorder.

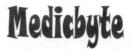

HISTORY AND COMMUNICATION 11

Advice to a pregnant woman-Instructions to candidates

This station tests your ability to advise a pregnant lady about the required investigations
- *A 39-year-old lady, Tina, is 14 weeks pregnant.*
- *She attends your prenatal clinic.*
- *She wishes to know what investigations that are appropriate for her and her baby as she is worried about her age affecting the pregnancy*

This station lasts for five minutes.

Now list the questions YOU will ask below:-

1..
....
2..
....
3..
....
4..
....
5..
....
6..
....
7..
....
8..
....
9..
....
10..
....

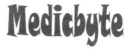

WHAT THE EXAMINER IS LOOKING FOR:-

CONSTRUCT

Educate the woman briefly about the necessary investigations and their significance.

OBJECTIVES

1. Communication
2. Brief history,
   of present pregnancy,
   past obstetric/ gynecology history.
   Specially ask about previous abnormal pregnancies , births or abortions,
   Abnormal births in the family.
3. Regular antenatal visits are necessary
   routine check ups,
   blood pressure
   obstetric examination
   weight check.
4. Blood group
   haemoglobin
   urinanalysis

5. Ultra sound is an investigation for foetal monitoring.

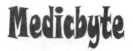

HISTORY AND COMMUNICATION 12

Dealing with a disruptive patient-Instructions to candidates

This station tests how you are going to deal with an aggressive patient on you ward

- *A 50-year-old man is going 'crazy' on the ward and he is being very abusive to nursing staff*
- *What necessary steps would you take to manage the situation?*

This station lasts for five minutes.

Now list the questions YOU will ask below:-

1...
....
2...
....
3...
....
4...
....
5...
....
6...
....
7...
....
8...
....
9...
....
10..
....

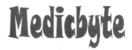

WHAT THE EXAMINER IS LOOKING FOR:-

CONSTRUCT

This is an emergency situation, you should be able to think of the important measures that should be taken, in order to stop any damage.

OBJECTIVES

1. Call the hospital security team
    Approach the patient in a non-confrontational manner
    Try to stop him, without hurting him
2. If this doesn't work, consider an intramuscular haloperidol.
3. Call hospital security team.
4. Look at present patient records to ascertain the level of danger likely.
5. Approach the patient in a non-confrontational manner.
6. Consider intramuscular haloperidol, however you must make sure that the patient is adequately restrained before approaching him. You will require one member of staff for each limb to hold him.

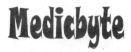

HISTORY AND COMMUNICATION 13

A case of peptic ulcer-Instructions to candidates

This station tests your ability to describe the condition simply to the patient

- *40 year old Mrs.Thomson has been diagnosed as having a peptic ulcer confirmed by endoscopy*
- *Counsel her about her condition and treatment briefly.*

This station lasts for five minutes.

Now list the questions YOU will ask below:-

1...
....
2...
....
3...
....
4...
....
5...
....
6...
....
7...
....
8...
....
9...
....
10...
....

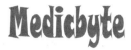

WHAT THE EXAMINER IS LOOKING FOR:-

CONSTRUCT

Simply explain the lady how she can make her condition better and what treatment she's going to get.

OBJECTIVES

1. Communication- introduce yourself
2. Tell her she has been diagnosed of peptic ulcer through history and investigations
   There is a defect in the lining of her duodenum.
3. The treatment is medical or surgical
   but surgery is undertaken only if there is a complication or medical treatment fails.
4. She will be given medicines i.e antacids,
   and other medication which will reduce the production of acid in the stomach
   (h2 antagnosists and proton pump inhibitors)
5. She will have to avoid
   smoking,alcohol
   Stress,
   Rich and oily food
   Take NSAIDS with care,
   Eat little after small intervals

Learning points

- In duodenal ulceration, the pain is in the epigastrium,
- Occurring when the patient is hungry - classically occurs at night.

- Important investigations include:

   Barium meal,
   Endoscopy to rule out carcinoma
   Acid secretion measurement OR
   serum gastrin in case of Zollinger Ellison syndrome.

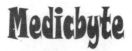

HISTORY AND COMMUNICATION 14:

Counselling a diabetic patient-Instructions to candidates

This station tests your ability to talk to a diabetic

- *55 year old Mr.Brown is a diabetic,he comes to your clinic for general advice*
- *Cousel him about his diet.*

This station lasts for five minutes.

Now list the questions YOU will ask below:-

1..
....
2..
....
3..
....
4..
....
5..
....
6..
....
7..
....
8..
....
9..
....
10..
....

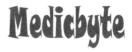

WHAT THE EXAMINER IS LOOKING FOR:-

CONSTRUCT

Make the patient understand what food should a diabetic have and what is not good for him.

OBJECTIVES

1. Communication
   brief introduction.

2. 'As he knows he has diabetes, he should learn about his dietary needs'.
   'He should avoid all forms of sugar or glucose',
   'That means avoiding all sweets including tinned fruits'.
   'All artificial drinks are high in sugar and should be avoided

3. He is also supposed to reduce fat intake and avoid oily foods.
   He can have foods and drinks made specially for diabetics with artificial sweeteners

4. Include fish,fresh vegetables and fruits in his diet.

Learning points

- Diabetics have to be careful about their diet whether they are on oral hypoglycemics or on insulin
- Daily calorie intake has to be monitored. They have to be aware of their dietary requirements themselves, which maintains a normal glucose level.
- Diabetics should undergo routine tests and examination by their doctor.

Diabetics learn, through a multidisciplinary approach, all aspects of their care. Regular follow up is necessary to ensure compliance.

The key word in complicated multi-system disorders is a **multidisciplinary approach**
Try to use this word in the examination.

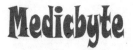

HISTORY AND COMMUNICATION 15

A case of varicose veins-Instructions to candidates

This station tests your ability to counsel a patient of varicose veins

- *60 year old,Mrs.Ralph has varicose veins, she has come to you*
- *Explain her what varicose veins are and how they are treated.*

This station lasts for five minutes.

Now list the questions YOU will ask below:-

1..
....
2..
....
3..
....
4..
....
5..
....
6..
....
7..
....
8..
....
9..
....
10..
....

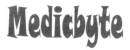

CONSTRUCT

Tell her what causes varicose veins and what is the treatment for them

OBJECTIVES

1. Communication
   introduce yourself
2. Varicose veins are dilated tortuous superficial veins in the legs
   they are caused because of a number of reasons,
      mainly due to dysfunction of the valves pumping blood from superficial to deep veins
      prolonged standing can aggravate the problem
3. There can be complications like thrombosis,
   ulceration
   skin changes
4. Prolonged standing should be avoided
   wear tight stockings for support,
   weight should be controlled,
   regular light exercise, like walking may be helpful
5. The permanent treatment for it is surgical.

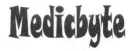

HISTORY AND COMMUNICATION 16

A case of chest pain-Instructions to candidates

This station tests your ability to take a relevant history to reach

- *A 65 year old man with a history of angina presents with chest pain*
- *The pain began 2 hours ago, it is a sharp pain not relieved by sublinginual nitrite therapy*

Ask the relevant questions to elicit the diagnosis

This station lasts for five minutes.

Now list the questions YOU will ask below:-

1..
....
2..
....
3..
....
4..
....
5..
....
6..
....
7..
....
8..
....
9..
....
10..
....

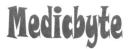

CONSTRUCT

As appropriate questions to elicit the cause of the pain, remembering that he has been on nitrite therapy

OBJECTIVES

1. Communication
   Introduce yourself
2. Ask about the pain (quality, onset, radiation, duration)
   Breathlessness
   Cold Sweats
   Pallor
   Previous attacks of angina
3. Past history of Strokes/TIA
   Past History of peripheral vascular disease (Hypertension, Diabetes)
   Oral contraceptive drugs
4. Family history of Myocardial infarctions, hypertension, diabetes
5. Risk Factors- smoking, occupation, eating habits lifestyle

Learning Points

This gentleman obviously has a history of angina and therefore his pain could be angina related, but the duration of this pain is long, and not relieved by medication. Therefore a myocardial infarction must be excluded.

Investigations
ECG- q wave changes and ST elevation
Cardiac Enzymes
CXR
ESR and White Cell Count are elevated

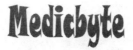

HISTORY AND COMMUNICATION 16

Consent for a procedure-Instructions to candidates

This station tests your ability to provide informed consent

- *A 40 year old man with acute appendicitis is about to go to surgery*
- *You are the surgical senior house officer on call*

Ask the relevant questions to elicit the diagnosis

This station lasts for five minutes.

Now list the questions YOU will ask below:-

1..
....
2..
....
3..
....
4..
....
5..
....
6..
....
7..
....
8..
....
9..
....
10..
....

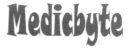

CONSTRUCT

You must provide detailed information to the patient without confusing him/her

OBJECTIVES

1. Communication
   Introduce yourself
2. Ask him/her if she/he knows about the operation and what will happen
   Answer questions appropriately
   Don't bluff if you don't know, tell him/her you will get back to him/her about a certain question if you cannot answer it
   Patients need sufficient information before they can decide to consent: for example
   Discuss the benefits and risks of the proposed treatment, and alternative treatments
   If the patient is not offered as much information, which they understand, as they reasonably need to make their decision, their consent may not be valid.
3. Questions regarding the general anaesthesia should be left for the anaesthetist
   Ask him/her if the anaesthetist has been to see her; if not offer to call the anaesthetist after your talk
   Oral contraceptive drugs

Key Points for consent

When do you need get consent?

1. Before you treat, examine or care for competent adult patient you must obtain consent.

2. Assume adults to be competent. If you are unsure about competence, ask yourself: "can this patient understand and weigh up the information needed to make this decision?" Unexpected decisions do not imply the patient is incompetent, but that further information or explanation may be needed.

3. Patients may be competent to make some health care decisions, even if they are not competent to make others.

4. Patients can change their minds and withdraw consent at any time. You should always check that the patient still consents to your caring for or treating them if you think that he/she may have changed her/his mind.

How do you consent children?

5. Like adults, before examining, caring or treating for a child, you must seek consent. Young people aged 16 to 17 are presumed to have the competence to give consent. Younger children who understand fully what is involved in the proposed procedure can also give consent (although their parents will ideally be involved). In other cases, some one with parental responsibility must give consent on the child's behalf, unless they cannot be reached in an emergency. If a competent child consents to treatment, a parent **cannot** over- ride that consent. Legally, a parent can consent if a competent child refuses, but it is likely that taking such a serious step will be rare.

Medicbyte

Who is the right person to get consent?

6. It is always best for the person actually treating the patient to seek the patient's consent.

You can get consent on behalf of colleagues if you are capable of performing the procedure in question, or if you have been specially trained to seek consent for the procedure.

Is the patient's consent voluntary?

7. Consent must be given voluntarily: not under any form of duress or undue influence from health professionals, family or friends.

Does it matter *how* the patient gives consent?

9. Consent can be written, oral or non- verbal. A signature on a consent form does not itself prove the consent is valid – the point of the form is to record the patient's decision, and also that discussions have taken place. Your hospital may have a policy setting out when you need to obtain written consent.

Refusals of treatment

10. Competent adult patients are entitled to refuse treatment, even where it would clearly benefit their health. The only exception to this rule is where the treatment is for a mental disorder and the patient is detained under the *Mental Health Act 1983* . A competent pregnant woman may refuse any treatment, even if this would be detrimental to the fetus.

Adults who are not competent to give consent

11. **No- one** can give consent on behalf of an incompetent adult. You may still treat such patients if the treatment would be in their best interests.

'Best interests' include factors such as the wishes and beliefs of the patient when competent, their current wishes, their general well- being and their spiritual and religious welfare as well as medical factors. People close to the patient may be able to give you useful information. Where the patient has never been competent, relatives, carers and friends may be best placed to advise on the patient's needs.

12. If an incompetent patient has clearly indicated in the past, while competent, that they would refuse treatment in certain circumstances ('ADVANCE REFUSAL'), and those circumstances arise, you must abide by that refusal.

Medicbyte

Medicbyte

Systematic Enquiry

Example Questions To Ask.

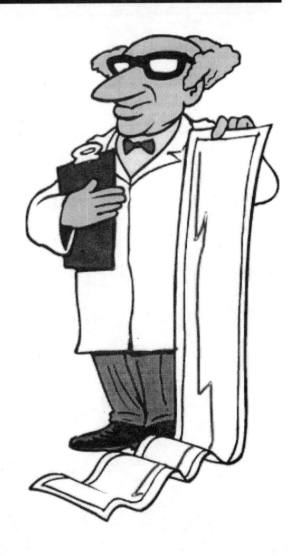

Medicbyte

Medicbyte

The history

The history provides you a way to get to know your patient and get as much information before undertaking the clinical examination.

These are the brief pieces of information you will need for a standard history. For the purposes of the PLAB you will have to tailor what you need depending on the case presented to you. Providing a tailored history is important in certain jobs such as accident and emergency.

NAME
AGE & DOB
OCCUPATION

PRESENTING COMPLAINT
HISOTY OF PRESENTING COMPLIANT
PAST MEDICAL HISTORY
DRUG HISTORY AND ALLERGIES
IMMUNISATION
FAMILY HISTORY
SOCIAL HISTORY

SYSTEMATIC ENQUIRY   This topic is addressed in detail in this chapter looking
                               at each of the systems

In the section that follows please remember the main questions for each organ system and also there are specific headings for special complaints that occur in the PLAB. You should the questions plus the specific questions to formulate an approach to each type of patient. Don't forget the time constraints in the examination. This section can never be complete because of the multitude of symptoms that can occur and candidates are encouraged to think on their toes and not to rely on rote memory when addressing clinical complaints. This section is only an example of the type of questions that you should consider.

Medicbyte

Pain....

Taking the history of pain is the bread and butter of medical history and so you should know to do this well.

Also you should get the patient to show you how and where the pain is and where it radiates.

- Onset   When did it start?
- Site   Where does it start?
- Character   What is it like?   Is it sharp like a knife cutting into you
                                    Is it a dull pain?
                                    Is it a band like pain?
- Severity of pain   Out of a score of 1 to 10 where 1 is no pain
                                    at all and 10 is the worst pain you can imagine;
                                    how bad is your pain
- How long does the pain last? Does it come and go?
- Radiation   Does the pain move to anywhere?
- Aggravating and relieving factors
- Associated symptoms   Do you sweat with the pain?
                                Palpitations- does your heart miss a beat or feel
                                as if it is beating differently?
                                When you have the pain do you get breathless

In the PLAB the following pain related scenarios may be present

- Pain points to a specific diagnoses or differential diagnosis. Here you will be expected to assimilate all the possible diagnoses and tell the examiner at the end of the consultation what you think.
- To manage a patients pain that he is currently having
- To alleviate the fear of pain of a patient with an oncological illness
                                (now about aspects of palliate care pain relief)

Good phrases and words to use to communicate effectively

One of the main aims of communication is not to offend the patient and so you should use words that are not derogatory, which have the desired meanings and patients can understand them. Examples are given below.

Back passage	The anal opening
Are your water works working properly?	To ensure micturation is OK
Have a bowel motion	
Have a pooh	To be used in children
Do you pass a lot of wind up the way or down the way?	This is a good way of asking About excessive flatulence or burping
Spit	Sputum
Overweight	Fat/Obese

Medicbyte

Gastrointestinal System

The gastrointestinal system gives ample opportunity for practice of the history and examination process. The PLAB 2 will test your ability to use words that are used in everyday practice by patients. You must be able to understand these to communicate effectively with patients. Examples are given in the table below.

Abdominal Pain	*Belly Pain*	
Bowels	Guts	
Bowel Motions	*Pooh*	
	Jobby	
Drugs	*Tablets*	
Mucous	*Slime*	
Pain	*Hurt*	
Patient points to sternum and describes a band like pain		Heart Burn
Passing Bowel Motions	*Poohing*	
Vomit	*Puke*	
Vomiting	*Puking*	

I have problems with vomiting doctor....

When did it start?
How long has it been going so far?
Is it worse if you do anything?
Is it relived if you do anything?
Do you also feel nauseas with it?
Is there blood in your vomit?
If yes, quantity and frequency
Is so how much blood would you say?
Is it worse with food?
Can drink OK?
Do you have problems swallowing food?
Have you had a high temperature?
Have you lost weight?
Do you have any other symptoms with it, like headache?
Do you make yourself vomit sometimes?
Do you take medications to make you vomit?
Other symptoms- abdominal pain, constipation, different abdomen, anorexia and vigilance
Headache (migraine, ICP, meningism).

Medicbyte

I have got pain in my belly, doctor....

Pain is a comon complaint and so you must know how to ask questions about this symptom.

Below are an example of questions you might ask.

Elicit the Character of Pain
- Is the pain a burning pain?
- Is the pain a heavy or crushing pain?
- Is the pain an aching pain?
- Is the pain a stabbing pain?
- Is the pain a sharp pain?
- Is the pain a dull ache?
- Is the pain gripping?

Frequency of the pain?
- How often does the pain come?
- Do you have spasms of pain?

Severity of the pain?
- Does the pain build up slowly?
- On a scale of 1 to 10 how bad is the pain?

Aggravating factors
- Is there anything, which makes the pain worse?
- Is there anything, which makes the pain better?

Associated symptoms
- When you have this pain do you have any other symptoms
  Such as- diarrhea, vomiting, sweating etc

Associated factors
- Does the pain come on after food? (gastritis/heartburn)
- Is the pain made worse on bending over? (hiatus hernia)

As you can see pain can be a complicated issue to work out. When attempting such a question remember the differential diagnosis of pain.

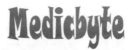

Diarrohea

When did it start?
What is the stool like? (hard, watery, formed, soft)
What colour is the stool? (same as usual; different)
Is there any blood in the stool?
Is there mucus (slime) in the stool?
How often are you passing stools?
Other symptoms- fever, vomiting, abdominal pain, weight loss

I am having difficulty swallowing doctor....

Is it painful when you swallow?
When did it start?
Is it getting worse, do you think?
Do you have difficulty with solids and liquids?
Do you feel food sticking in your throat?
If you do feel food sticking, please point to where you think it is the worst?

(Patient may point to his chest)

Have you lost any weight?
Has anyone complained that you have got bad breathe?
Apart from the difficulty in swallowing; do you also suffer from vomiting?
If you vomit; do you see food in your vomit? (implies incomplete digestion)

Jaundice

Who first noticed your colour change?
Or when did you notice your skin go yellow?
Did the yellowness get worse quickly?
Has the yellowness got any better?
Does the colour change; get better and then worse?

Do you also get pain in you belly, if so where?   Pain may be present in the right hypochondrium

Have you lost your appetite?
What colour is your urine?
What colour are the bowel motions?
Have you had any recent blood transfusions?
Have you had any injections recently?

Some people who get this problem may have had many needle injections in the past? (*You are trying to probe the possibility of IV drug abuse). Remember don't be too blunt in the examination; try to remain courteous at all times.*

Have you been in contact with anyone who also has had the same problem?
Are you finding yourself getting very thirsty?

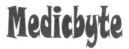

Alcohol History

Do you drink?
How often do you drink?
Then you should ask the CAGE questions

Cut   Have you felt you should cut down on Drinking?
Annoy   Have you annoyed anyone (family, friends) with your drinking?
Guilt   Have you felt guilty about your drinking?
Eye Opener   Have you had alcohol as an 'eye opener' first thing in the morning?

What to do with problem drinkers…..

Services are available in the UK that will help support patients with drinking problems. Your emphasis should be to identify at risk patients and then to counsel them on how they can seek help.

Alcohol rehabilitation centers
Alcoholics Anonymous   These are groups where people with alcohol related
Problems meet. There is one group facilitator who
Counseling skills. The emphasis is on sharing
Experiences with others and using group dynamics
To solve drink related problems.

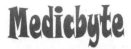

Blood Per Rectum….

You say you have seen blood coming from your back passage?

When did this start? Or When did you first notice this?

You say blood, what colour is it?   Red
                                                                   Deep red

Does it look like fresh blood? Or does it look more like old blood?

This question helps to differentiate Melaena from fresh blood

Do you also see mucous in the stool?

Are the stools normal or are they very runny?

This is to elicit whether there is diarrhea with the symptoms

When does the blood come from your back passage?

If the patient doesn't know what you are talking about then follow on with the question below...

Do you find that the blood is seen when you go to the toilet to have a bowel motion?

If he/she says that yes it does come at the time of a bowel motion then ask….

Do you see blood at the beginning, middle or end of a bowel motion?

Do you feel like going to the toilet many times during the day? For example when you are out shopping?

Do you get pain with the blood?

Are you stools normally easy to flush away and does the toilet paper you use feel fatty?

Do you pass a lot of wind up the way or down the way?

When you have finished passing the bowel motion does it ever feel as if you haven't quite passed all of the motion?

Does anyone in the family have similar complaints?

If the complaint started recently then pursue diarrhea history...

Have you been abroad recently?
                         Other related questions

Has your appetite been OK?

Have you lost any weight?

Have you eaten anything differently recently?

Have you been on any medication, for example have you been taking medicine that thins your blood?

Medicbyte

Cardiovascular System

Questions for the cardiovascular system are straightforward. What confuses students is the fact that the cardiovascular system and the respiratory system are inherently linked.

Breathlessness
Palpitations-   Are you aware of your heartbeat?
                                                   Do you have an irregular heart beat (tap your fingers to
                                                   show the patient)
                                                   Do you think your heart beat is fast or slow?
Dyspnea –Orthopnea   Does the breathlessness get worse on lying down?
                                                   Can you lie flat at night, if not how many pillows
                                                   Do you use?
Paroxysmal Nocturnal Dyspnea   Do you suddenly wake up at night
                                                   finding it difficult to breathe?
Swelling (dependant oedema)   Do you suffer from swelling of your limbs; worse
                                                   at the end of the day?
                                                   Do the rings on your fingers get tight?
                                                   Are your eyelids swollen or puffy in the morning?
                                                   Can you fit into your shoe at the end of your day?

Breathlessness
Tiredness
Intermittent claudication   Do you have pain in your calves
                                                   and how far can you walk?
                                                   Is it relived when you rest?
Cough   Do you have a cough?
                                                   Are you on any medicines for your heart? ACEI Cough
Haemoptysis (pulmonary oedema)   Have you coughed up blood
Signs of arterial insufficiency   Do your muscles ache (especially thigh/calf)
Signs of venous insufficiency   Do you develop swelling in your legs
                                                   at the end of the day?
                                                   Do you have any varicose veins or ulcers in your legs?

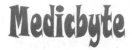

Chest Pain

The usual pain questions (see previous) are to be used to tease out the possible diagnoses.
When questioning the patient with chest pain consider the differential diagnosis which given below.

Myocardial Infarction	Central chest pain that can radiate to the jaw and arm Lasts more than 30 minutes, present at rest Not relieved by nitrates Associated with sweating/nausea and vomiting
Angina	Less severe than the above pain Associated with exertion Lasts less than 30 minutes Relived by nitrates (there are variations in the presentation and types of angina)
Pericarditis	Retro-sternal pain, worse on inspiration/lying down. Relieved by sitting forward. There may be a pericardial rub.
Pericardial effusion	
Dissecting aneurysm	Retrosternal sharp pain radiating to the back
Pleurisy	Pain worse on deep inspiration, patients say that it catches their breathe
Pneumothorax	Sudden sharp pain
Thoracic disc prolapse	Pain may positional; other associated Neurological signs may be present
Oesphageal reflux/gastritis	Burning retro-sternal chest pain Patient describes a band-like vertical pain
Muscloskeletal pain	See the joints section

Heart Failure

New York Heart Association Classification of Heart failure in terms of function of everyday activity

Grade 1 No limitation in any action
Grade 2 No limitation of daily activity, but symptoms occur on everyday exertion
Grade 3 Everyday activity limited by symptoms
Grade 4 All activity is very limited; patient is chair bound or bed bound

How many steps can you get up before having to stop?
Can you do your own shopping?
How far can you walk before getting breathless?
Can you do the housework?
What can't you do now which you could do in the past?

Medicbyte

Respiratory System

Breathlessness	
Cough	
Haemoptysis	See below
Chest pain	
Sputum	Do you cough anything up?
	If so what colour is it?
Smoking history	Do you smoke?
Occupational History	welder- occupational asthmatic
	Farmer- farmers lung
Pet's	Pigeon- pigeon fancier disease

Wheeze

Do you find it difficult to breathe?
What happens?
Can you hear a noise when you breathe, a wheeze?
Do you also have problems with a cough?
What makes the wheeze better?
What makes the wheeze worse?
Do you have pets in the house?
Do you have dusty bed sheets?
Do you or anyone in the house smoke?
Do you exercise regularly?
Is the wheeze worse in the cold weather?
Is the wheeze worse when you have a cold?

Haemoptysis

Have you coughed up blood?

How often does it happen?

Has it got better, or has it got more frequent?

When did it start?

Is it associated with bouts of coughing?

If so how many teaspoons do you cough up every time?

Do you smoke? If so, how many cigarettes do you smoke a day?

Have you lost weight?

Do you suffer from any other illnesses?

Medicbyte

Cough

Cough is a complex symptom, the pointer to a long differential diagnosis.

The aim of a cough consultation would be to elucidate the cause, so first think differential diagnosis.

Once you have a differential diagnosis in your head you can ask the correct type of questions.

ASK ABOUT THE COUGH and then go through the list below

Smoking history/cancer
How many cigarettes do you smoke a day?
How many years have you been smoking for?
Have you lost weight?
Have you coughed up any blood?

Asthma/Atopy
Nighttime cough
Cough bought on by exercise
Cough aggravated by dust/pollen/recent colds/painting/renovation of the house
No weight loss
Ask about medication- may be on long term inhalers
Ask about other allergies and also ask about eczema
Ask about family history

Chronic Bronchitis
Chronicity
Sputum
Smoking history

Tuberculosis
Chronic cough
Nighttime sweats
Ethnic origin
Weight loss

Heart failure
Breathlessness
Paroxysmal Nocturnal Dyspnea
Ask other cardiovascular related questions

Medicbyte

Neurological System

Headache

What time of day?
What type of pain is it?
When did it begin?
How bad is it? Is the pain the worse you ever had?
Do you have any problems with your eyesight? Do you wear glasses?
Photophobia-   Are you irritable to light?
Meningism   Are you suffering from neck stiffness
Do you feel nauseous?
Where is the headache (unlateral/bilateral/temporal/frontal/occiptial)

> Temporal headache- temporal arteritis
> Occipital- sub arachnoid haemorrhage
> Frontal- sinusitis

Do you problems with weakness in your limbs
Do you suffer from fits?
Are you taking any medicines?
Is there a family history of migraine?
Are there any foods that bring on the headache?
Are there any problems at work? Do you have any stresses, such as marital etc
Do you take any medicines to make the pain better?

Associated systems   Power loss (e.g. tumour)
                         Squints

Loss of consciousness

When does it occur?
What are the aggravating factors?
Do you suffer form epilepsy?
How do you feel when you are about to have these episodes?
Does anyone else in your family suffer from such problems?
Do you remember the events afterwards?
How long does it take for you to come around?
Is it associated with long periods of standing?
Did you have a knock to your head a few days ago?

Vision

Medicbyte

How is you eyesight? Do you wear glasses?
The problems with your eyesight; did it get worse slowly or did it happen suddenly?

Long-sighted or Shortsighted	Do you have problems with looking at things far away or do you have problems with close objects?
Ask about the visual field	Is the whole of your field of vision affected or only a part of it?
Ask about Scotomas	Are there spots or specks in the visual field? Do the specks move around?

Specks/spots that move = floaters in the vitreous

Scotomas are fixed defects= retinal or visual pathway lesions

Conjuctivitis	Is your eye painful? Have the eyes been red, if so how long? Did the redness in the eyes begin in one eye, both eyes or one eye then the next? Has your eyelid been sore? When you open and close your eye does it hurt?
Adequate lacrimation	Can you close your eyelids fully? Are you eyes always watery?
Diplopia Horizontal diplopia Vertical Diplopia	Do see double vision? If so are the images alongside each-other; next to each other or above and below each other

Medicbyte

Medicbyte

The Clinical Examination And Practical skills

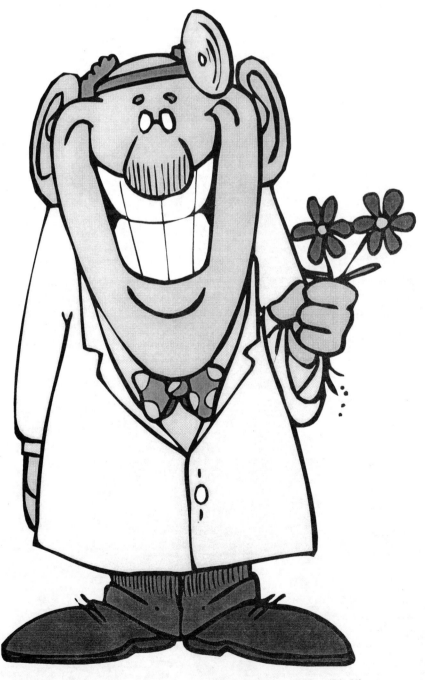

Medicbyte

Medicbyte

The OSCE examination

The OSCE part of the examination tests your *basic skills at clinical examination*. The GMC are not looking for you to pick up amazing signs, but that you have a good basic approach to clinical examination.

This section is divided into two. The clinical examination section and the procedures section. Ideas of classical examination technique are further illustrated by MEDICBYTE Videos that are available separately.

CLINICAL EXAMINATION

Undertake the medical examination of any system including Musculoskeletal examination
Rectal or bimanual vaginal examination
Assess limps and bumps in males and females and offer a differential diagnosis
Be able to assess a peak flow
Be able to measure blood pressure
Mental state examination
You should be comfortable with the use of an ophthalmoscope or auriscope
You may be asked to write down your findings (include time, date, name of patient and signed by your full name)

This can be a stressful station because not only must you complete the objectives but you must also do so in a respectful manner. This will be achieved through practice.

Reviews in the following type of patients

(1)   Diabetic
(2)   Asthmatic
(3)   Cystic Fibrosis
(4)   Sickle cell
(5)   Rheumatoid arthritis

CLINICAL PROCEDURES

Procedures that you should know about

Assessment of Glasgow Coma Score
Venous cannulation and setting up an IV bag
Landmarks for central venous access
Lumbar puncture
Male catherisation
Cervical smear

Cardiopulmonary resuscitation

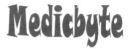

The Culture Shock- time constraints

Coming from India I have come to realize the change in cultural attitudes that are expected when you come to work in the UK.

I was used to seeing a high volume of patients whilst undertaking government practice India; this meant that I could spend very little time with them.

Therefore in India my questioning was very direct and to the point.

I had to take on a different attitude to pass the PLAB 2 here in the UK. I also learnt what you do in the PLAB 2 is the ideal examiners wish for you to attain. Even in UK practice time is a limitation and it is sometimes not possible to spend as much time with patients as I would wish.

However as the OSCE stations have a time limit it helps you to think on your feet and not to forget the important details.

Dr K Patel

Medicbyte

Section One

Clinical Examination

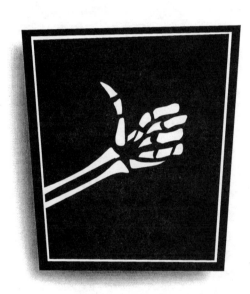

**'On preparing for the
Clinical Examination remember you
really only have five minutes
on the day per station!!'**

Medicbyte

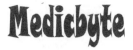

Clinical Examination

There is no doubt that CLINICAL EXAMINATION is vital to you if you are practising as a doctor.

The aim of examiners in testing clinical examination is to

1. Ensure you are courteous and considerate to the patients.
2. Do not inflict pain on.
3. Have a standard approach that is clinically sound.
4. Don't miss doing important actions, e.g. peak flow.
5. Keeps to time (4 and a half minutes)

Just remember the basics and be well rehearsed so that by the time the examination comes along you look as though you have done the task asked 'a hundred times'.

This section on Clinical Examination is only an aide memoir of what is needed for the examination. For further detailed explanation on clinical examination please refer to the recommended textbooks on the Medicbyte Website.

We will not emphases this further within the chapter, but BE COURTEUOS. When the examiner asks you to do something don't just jump into the examination.

Medicbyte Courtesy Tips:-

1. Introduce Yourself
2. Ensure patient Privacy (curtains drawn/ doors closed)
3. Explain to the patient what you are about to do
4. Ensure that you do not inflict pain (keep an eye on the patient)

Do you talk to the examiner or not?

My personal opinion is that you should practice as though you will be expected to talk to the examiner describing every step of what you are doing. As there is a strict time constraint your examination and your descriptions need to be concise and slick so as not to bore the examiner and not to waste time.

If the examiner asks you to keep quiet and to describe your findings at the end; then that should be straightforward if you have learnt to talk through examinations; you can easily keep quiet.

Time constraints.......

The time constraints are a major problem limiting the level of patient interaction. So your systems examination must be slick; to the point.

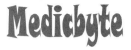

HOW I PRACTICED CLINICAL EXAMINATION- The MEDICBYTE Minds Eye Approach'

I was finding it hard to practice the full examination on all my patients all the time. I therefore decided to practice in my 'minds eye'. I learnt this technique for a sports psychologist.

Every-day I would spend time thinking about the examination and what it would be like and imagined my-self in the examination being examined.

The examiner would ask me; please Dr Roberts, examine the respiratory system. I would then in my minds eye go through every step of the examination process. I would talk to the examiner as if he was real and I made sure I did not miss any step out in the examination.

At the same time as doing this I would practice on a make believe patient (my teddy bear). Also I would think up common clinical situations; e.g. the acute abdomen or consolidation and I would know what to sat for each possible differential.

In this way by the time of the examination I had practiced more than I could have ever imagined, on the day of the examination I managed to do my clinical cases quickly, I didn't annoy the examiner and I passed!

The purpose of the PLAB clinical examination is to ensure that you have a good clinical technique. Although some patients will have detectable pathology others will not.

The examiner wishes to ensure that:-

1. You have a logical approach to clinical examination
2. You are sensitive to your patients wishes
3. You communicate well with the patent
4. You can present you findings

Doctors misjudge how much weight point 2 carries in the examination process. So even if you are nervous, think about your patient and do not seem discourteous even if you don't mean to be.

In the PLAB 2 course held my medicbyte there are many mannerisms or approaches to patients, which we as teachers have to rectify in the students.

We therefore suggest it a good idea if your technique is analysed by an experienced examiner.

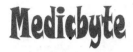

Acting Out the Stations

The problem with clinical examinations is that they take doctors out of context from the clinical situation and you are expected to perform in a certain time period for examiners.

This is artificial because medical education is an ongoing process. Doctor also do make mistakes and the good ones learn from them.

For the PLAB 2 the aim is to make mistakes before the examination during practice sessions; courses are available and the Medicbyte course for the PLAB 2 provides experienced clinicians to teach you.

An important tip that I will give you is that you should think of yourself as actors acting out scenes in a play. Certain aspects of how you examine, how you greet the patient, how you undertake skill tasks should be exaggerated. Exaggeration allows you to tell the examiner that you know what you should be doing and look I am doing it.

For example when placing a sharp into a sharps bin; do so carefully, slowly, precisely and make use of hand actions.

Don't irritate the examiner with a snails pace drop of the sharps needle into the sharps bin.

Another tip I give to students is watch and learn from actors in medical soaps that appear on TV- you should be trying to emulate the good doctors on these programs in how they handle the patients and how they appear so confident in front of the camera.

Medicbyte

Medicbyte

Neurology

'Examine this mans cranial nerves'

Sometimes the examiner will be more specific, especially if time is of the essence and then specific questions like 'examine the seventh nerve' or 'examine the facial nerve'. So you should know how to examine specific nerves.

Cranial nerves   I   Olfactory

> *'Do you have any problems with smell'*

II   Optic

> Visual acuity
> Colour vision
> Visual field
> Direct and Consensual light reflex reflexes
> Examine Fundus

III   Occulomotor

> Test Eye Movements
> Look for ptosis

IV   Trochlear
> Test Eye Movements
> (superior oblique)

V   Trigeminal
> Light touch to the three divisions of the facial nerve
> *'Grin clenching your teeth'*(masseter)
> *'Move the jaws sibeways'*(the pterygoids)
> Jaw Jerk
> Corneal/Conjunctival Reflexes

VI   Abducent
> Eye Movements
> (lateral rectus)

Medicbyte

VII   **Facial**
Look for deviation of the face
Widened palpebral fissure
Loss of nasolabial fold
Ask the patient :
Frown
Close your eyes tightly
Smile or show your teeth
Blow your mouth
Taste on anterior two thirds of tongue

VIII   **Vestibulocochlear**
Two components:
Vestibular:
Test for nystagmus
Vertigo
Chochlear:
Tests for deafness:
Rinne's test
Weber's test
Absolute bone conduction test

IX   **Glossophrayngeal**

Taste on posterior one third of toungue(usually difficult)
Elicit gag reflex.

X   **Vagus**
Observe the voice(look for nasal quality)
Ask the patient :
Say aah
Note the movement of uvula(it moves towards the normal side in
unilateral lesions
palatal/pharangeal reflexes
if dysphonia(vocal cords should be inspected)

XI   **Accessory**
Check sternomastoids:
Look for any wasting
Ask the patient :
Press your chin down(against resistance)
Turn your head sideways(against resistance)
Check the trapezius:
Look for wasting
Ask the patient:
Shrug your shoulders(against resistance)

XII   **Hypoglossal**
Examine movements of the tongue.
Look for tremors/fasciculation
On protruding out the tongue deviates toward the paralysed side

Medicbyte

Medicbyte

Neurology

COMMAND:

'Examine this Gentleman's' arms/Legs'

PREREQUISITES:
Introduce yourself
Obtain consent
Expose properly
Remember to compare both sides

STEPS:

INSPECTION
Look for:
Wasting
Fasciculations

PALPATION

Bulk
Compare both limbs

Tone
Equal, Reduced, Increased
Or hyper/hypotonia
Power
Reduced, Power
Grade Power(0-5)

Reflexes
Know the Reflex root values
Know the pattern of loss for the main medical conditions (Upper motor Neurone, Lower Motor Neurone)

Sensation
Tests for sensory function:
Touch
Pain(don't hurt the patient){superficial and deep)
Temperature
Proprioception
Vibration
Cortical localisation-2 point discrimination
                -steriognosis
                -graphesthesia
(You should know the dermatomes on the limbs and check sensations accordingly)
Coordination
Look at specific function
Know
The different patterns of neurological deficit
You must be proficient in the examination of the system; knowing minuscule detail of neurological conditions is not needed (you are not doing a neurologists examination)
The neurological and Cardiovascular systems are the most important to know for the PLAB II

Medicbyte

COMMAND

Examine the cerebellar functions

PREREQUISITES
Introduce yourself
Obtain consent
Expose where needed

STEPS

Carry out tests for the following in this sequence:

NYSTAGMUS
Do not ask the patient to focus too far or too close or laterally

SPEECH
Look for Dysarthria
Slurred speech

SPECIFIC TESTS
Finger-nose test
Finger-finger test
Heel-knee-shin test
Look for intention tremors
Past pointing
Dysdiadochokinesia

REFLEX
Pendular knee jerk

GAIT
Typical drunken(staggering)gait
Ataxia

Medicbyte

Gastrointestinal System

COMMAND

'Examine this lady's abdomen'

PREREQUISITES

Introduction
Obtain consent
Expose properly
(ideal exposure for abdominal examination is from nipples to mid thighs)

STEPS

INSPECTION
Inspect carefully
Note down the findings
Scars,
Veins,
Abdominal shape
Hernias
Resp movements
Pulsations
Peristalsis
Examination of genitalia

PALPATION
Look for tenderness

Warning!!
Remember to look at the patient as you are examining because if the patient winces with pain and
You do not notice you will be marked down.
Guarding
Palpate liver,(span of liver)
Spleen and
Kidneys
Abdominal masses
Hernial orifices
Fluid thrill if you suspect fluid
Inguinal lymph nodes
Rectal examination should be done with every abdominal examination

PERCUSSION

The abdominal organs(liver and spleen)
The percussion note(fluid or gas)
Shifting dullness(if abdomen is protuberant)

AUSCULTATION
Bowel sounds
Vascular bruits

Medicbyte

Respiratory System
COMMAND

'Examine this man's chest'

PREREQUISITES

Introduction
Obtain consent
Expose properly from front and back

STEPS

INSPECTION
Note down the findings
Shape
Movements with respiration
Mode of respiration
The usual findings like scars,
Pulsations
Pigmentation

PALPATION
Tenderness
subcutaneous emphysema
Position of trachea
Chest expansion/movement
Vocal fremitus

PERCUSSION
Anterior posterior and lateral chest wall
Hepatic dullness
Cardiac dullness

AUSCULTATION
Auscultate for breath sounds
Added sounds
Vocal resonance

Medicbyte

Cardiovascular System

COMMAND
'Auscultate the heart'

PREREQUISITES

Introduction
Obtain consent
Expose the chest properly

STEPS IN AUSCULTATION

Follow the same pattern
Make a habit of inspecting before touching the patient

For auscultation:
Palpate for apex beat
Localize it

AUSCULTATION
Place your stethoscope on the mitral area(at the apex) and listen carefully
Move to tricuspid area(4th intercostals space at the left sternal edge)
Then to pulmonary (2nd intercostal space at the left strenal edge)
Aortic area(2nd intercostals space at the right sternal edge)

Take time to listen to the heart sounds and notice any added sounds
What are the heart sounds like? Is the first heart sound present and is the second heart sound present
Are they soft or loud,is the second heart sound split?(normal on inspiration)
For detailed auscultation for murmurs

Medicbyte

Aortic stenosis
Ejection systolic murmur
Maximal in 2nd LICS
Radiating into neck and apex

Pulmonary stenosis
mid-systolic murmur
Maximal in2nd LICS

Aortic regurgitation
Early diastolic murmur
Maximal in 3rd LICS or less often in 2nd RICS
Make the patient sit and bend forward,ask him to breathe in and out and hold it.
Listen with the diaphragm over the aortic area.

Pulmonary regurgitation
Early diastolic murmur
Maximal in 2nd and 3rd LICS

Mitral stenosis
mid diastolic murmur
loud 1st sound
opening snap
presystolic accentuation of murmur
turn patient to left
or make him sit and bend forward
Listen with the bell of the stethoscope

Mitral regurgitation
Pan-systolic at apex
Radiates to axilla

VSD
Pan systolic
Maximal at 3rd 4th LICS parasternally

ASD
Pulmonary systolic murmur with fixed split 2nd sound

PDA
Machinery murmur (heard through first and second heart sounds)
Heard best in 2nd 3rd LICS in mid-clavicular line

Aortic Coarctation
Loud murmur in systole
Maximal over apex of left lung also look for FRICTION RUB

Medicbyte

SURGICAL CASES

COMMAND

' Examine the swelling over this man's cheek'

PREREQUISITES

Introduction
Obtain consent
Make the view clear by moving the head of the patient

STEPS

INSPECTION
On inspection, keep in mind the following points:
Site of the swelling
Size,
Shape,
Extent
Overlying skin

PALPATION
Tenderness (ask the patient if it hurts)
Surface
Consistency
Edges
Margins
Temperature of overlying skin
Relation with underlying structures(fixed or mobile)
Relation to overlying skin
Always remember to palpate the draining lymph nodes

PERCUSSION
Not required
Maybe required for large, non-tender swellings

AUSCULTATION
Not usually required
Just in specific conditions like goitre to look for bruit.

Medicbyte

COMMAND

' *Examine the ulcer on the man's foot.* '.

PREREQUISITES

Communication.
Obtain consent
Proper exposure.

STEPS

INSPECTION

Look for:
Site,
Shape,
Extent,
Floor,
Base,
Edges,
Margins
Adjacent structures.

PALPATION

Tenderness,
Any discharge(fluid or pus)
Draining lymph nodes

Medicbyte

COMMAND

'Examine this woman's right breast.'

PREREQUISITES

Communication
Obtain consent
Expose properly

STEPS

INSPECTION

Examine both breasts.
The inspection is carried out in three steps:
Arms by the side,
Hands placed on the hips
Arms above the head
Things to be looked for:

SKIN:
Any visible deformity,
Any swelling,
Ulcer,
Any dimpling of skin(specially with arms above the head)
AREOLA
Any ulcer
Cracking
NIPPLES
Everted or inverted
Any discharge
If present,type,colour and smell
If blood is present in the discharge

PALPATION

Examine both breasts,
Start with the normal breast.
Palpate with the plm of the hand keeping it straight
Feel for any nodules,
If present notice the site,
Size
Consistency
Mobility
Check if it is fixed to the chest wall (by asking the patient to press her hand on the hip) and then move it,if it does not move it means it is fixed to the chest wall.
Examine the lymph nodes(axillary and supraclavicular)

Medicbyte

Managing Common Conditions in the UK

For The PLAB Examination

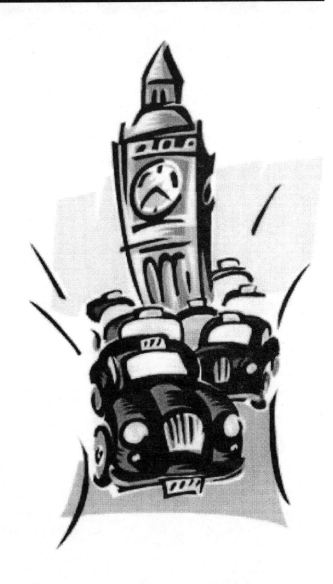

Medicbyte

Medicbyte

You will be expected to have some knowledge of the management of some important and very common conditions for the PLAB. You do not need to go into tremendous detail but you should have a feel for these conditions so that in however they are presented to you in the examination you can attempt to manage your patient.

Also remember there is a psychological impact to the every disease process and you should be sensitive to this.

In managing clinical conditions examiners test your ability to:-

Explain diagnoses to patients
Explain the ongoing disease process
Help the patient understand the impact of the disease on lifestyle
Help the patient make lifestyle choices for disease modulation
Explain the different drugs for a condition and who they work
Assess compliance of medication or to certain life style choices (e.g. giving up smoking)
Reassure patients and parents

In this section we have provided you with two examples of conditions.
During your work up to the PLAB look at other examples. Remember that often these conditions seldom occur in the same frequency in the host countries of PLAB candidates so be sure to learn up on these conditions.

Medicbyte

Medicbyte

Management Of Crohns Disease

Crohns disease is a favourite of UK examination systems because of its effects; the challenge in diagnosis through history and examination, and the ongoing management issues.

Diagnosis	History	
	Examination	
	Investigations	What is the extent of the disease?
		Upper bowel: Barium follow-through
		Lower bowel: Colonscopy and ileoscopy

Monitoring Disease Activity

Is the disease affecting the body?   Weight parameters (weight loss)

Are there any complications of Crohns disease?
          Intestinal obstruction- Abdominal X-ray

Intra abdominal abscess- radiolabelled white cells

Transabdominal ultrasound- abscess/fistulae detection

Abdominal CT- abscess/fistulae detection/perianal complications

Treatment

Counseling-	Be able to explain to a patient what is meant by the diagnosis? Be able to explain the investigations/treatments/management of the condition
Support	Know about relevant support agencies- National Association for Colitis and Crohn's disease
Diet	elemental diets may be used to induce remission
Drugs-	Antidiarrheal drugs Cholestyramine Vitamins and Minerals
	Corticosteroids New 5-aminosalicylates Flagyl/Ciprofloxacin for active Crohns
	Immunosupression Anitumour necrosis factor alpha antibody
	Avoid NSAIDS if possible
Surgery	Surgery is not curative Balloon dilatation of strictures

Medicbyte

Management Of Asthma

Asthma again is ideal for UK examinations. Below are a list of typical questions…

Talk to some one about the diagnosis?

Asthma is like an allergy; except it affects your airways. If the allergy is severe your airways narrow and you find it difficult to breathe. The good news is that in between times your lungs are fine. Different people have different levels of narrowing, if it is out of control then you will need lots of medicine, however some people only have minimal problems with it.

What is the management of the condition?

There are a number of ways of helping yourself to help you stay healthy if you have asthma. There are things you can do (lifestyle choices) and there are things that we can do to help (drug management).

Lifestyle choices?

Staying healthy is very important in helping you body. There are certain type of exercises that you can do to help you lungs these are swimming or jogging. Smoking is not good for your lungs and avoiding things that make your asthma worse is also a good idea.

Manage an acute asthma attack in an emergency?

Manage an asthmatic in terms of long-term medications?

Know about the medications used in the management of an asthma attack….

Medicbyte

Section Two

Practical Procedures

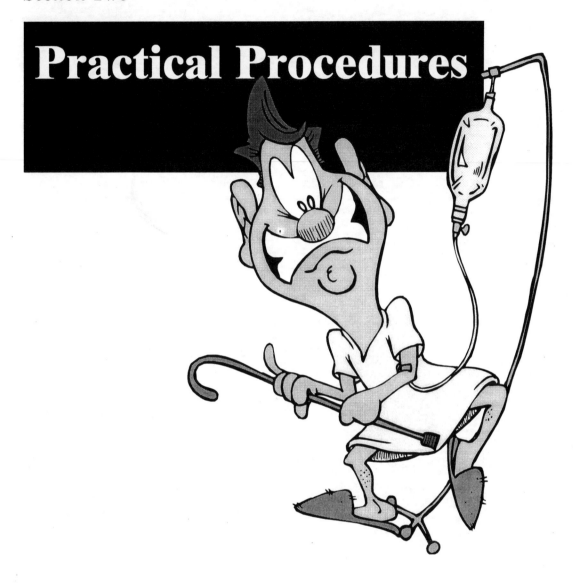

Medicbyte

Medicbyte

Practical skills for the PLAB examination: a suggested approach

A suggested method for tackling procedures in the examination is given below. It is important that for anything that you do in the examination, and in 'real' clinical practice, that you have devised a method for most things. This is because it is in the moments of tiredness or stress that clinical errors occur. Error is something that our patients cannot afford.

1. Tell your patient what you are going to do, put the patient at ease

2. Prepare what you will need for the procedure, ensuring an aseptic approach

3. Undertake the procedure ensuring you sensitivity to the patient

4. Make sure you take care and clean up the utensils at the end

5. Make a clear statement at the end of the procedure to inform your patient that the procedure is over and what he/she must do (e.g. Lumbar puncture- *'lie flat on your back for a few hours'*.

To practice the methods and skills required for the PLAB part 2 you can attend courses and practise at home on your partner or any other willing assistant. Various courses allow you to practise on manikins and models and take you through the steps of an OSCE type of examination. Please contact the Medicbyte team at plab@medicbyte.com to find about a PLAB course near to your examination.

'don't forget to pull the blinds'

Even if you are examining dummies make a point of ensuring privacy- pull the blinds and tell the examiner:-

- I will ensure privacy for the patient at all times
- I will ensure that the patient is informed about everything I will do
- If the patient does not wish for me to continue I will stop and after talking to the patient stop the procedure if necessary; I will record this in the notes

Various practical procedures are discussed in this section. Try to practice these in your spare time. Using clinical models can be a good way of getting proficient in these skills. Such models are available at the Medicbyte PLAB 2 course.

Rectal and vaginal examinations are discussed in the PLAB 2 videos by Medicbyte.

Medicbyte

Medicbyte

PLAB Procedure one

Venous cannulation/ Venepuncture

In an era of HIV and blood borne disease needle-stick safety is of paramount importance to you, your patients and fellow colleagues. This procedure if done well should not hurt the patient. Also know what tests are needed or the level of difficulty of venflon placement. When you know what tests are required you can get the relevant bottles ready. If you know that venous cannulation is going to be difficult then you should call a more experienced colleagues after three goes.

1.   Tell your patient what you are going to do, put the patient at ease

'Hello Mrs...I need to take a blood sample from you'.

'Hello Mr...we need to put a venflon into your arm/hand so that we can give you fluids (or antibiotics) directly into your veins'.

2.   Ask the patient if he/she has any bleeding problems

'Do you suffer from any bleeding or clotting disorders?'

3.   Prepare what you will need for the procedure, ensuring an aseptic approach

This is what you will need

Venepunture	**Intravenous devise**
Gloves	Gloves
Sharps bin	Sharp bin
Needle	venflon
Syringe/blood letting suction application	Fixing tape/plaster
Torniquet	Torniquet
Cotton wool	Cotton wool
Plaster	
Specimen bottles and forms	

4.   Identify a suitable vein- time taking here will save you time later

Medicbyte

5.   Undertake the procedure ensuring your you are sensitive to your patient's feelings

Use a tourniquet (it is a good idea for you to carry your own and use it an as many arms as possible so that you don't fumble in the examination).

'I am just going to put his torniquet around you and tighten it, this will help your veins stand up'

So doctors find that tapping on the vein makes it stand up
'I am just going to make your veins stand up'

'You don't have to look if you don't want to'

'You will feel a scratch and then the procedure will be completed. Some people find that it is better to look away'.

Using your left hand if you are right handed and vice versa, support the patients arm/hand whilst pulling the skin taut while with the dominant hand place the needle or venflon.
For the needle

Withdraw blood

For the venflon

You may see a flash back of blood coming into your cannula and as you advance the plastic sheath of the venflon withdraw the needle slowly from the plastic sheath.

6.   Make sure you take care and clean up the utensils

Medicbyte

Important Rules

AVIOD INFECTED AREAS OR ODEMATOUS AREAS

LABEL HIGH RISK SAMPLES WITH BIO HAZARD LABELS

NEVER RESEATH A USED NEEDLE; instead place it straight in the sharps bin after use.

Know the sharps Injury policy for your hospital

Sharps Bins

Characteristically these are yellow in colour and you should ensure that the sharps bin lid is on properly. Also never over fill a sharps bin. Know what must always go in a sharps bin and what can go as 'ordinary' hospital disposal. Generally anything that is sharp or has been contaminated with body fluid must go into a sharps bin. Nappies etc go into hospital waste.

Some bins have a slot where the needles can be fed to and gripped.

Vacutainer systems

You should know the different methods of blood letting and something that is very popular in the UK is the vacu-container system. This system provides filling of spaceman bottles directly from the patient's arm without the need of a syringe. Only one puncture of the vein is required using a special devise which allows bottles to be placed on it and filled directly.

The bottle colour coding used in UK hospitals is similar, you should know for your hospital roughly which investigation goes in which bottle.

Sharps Injuries

Every UK hospital has sharps injury policy which basically involves the following:-

Wash immediately
Report to occupational health
Remember to document the injury

What to do with the blood samples

In real clinical practice you will be expected to safely label each sample and place it into a plastic bag with a slip detailing the request. High-risk samples (Hepatitis B or HIV) samples should be placed in a bag with a 'danger' sign on it. In the request form of a HIV patient some doctors do not write 'IV infection' but instead T4 deficiency in an attempt to provide some form of dignity to the patient and not to frighten staff handling the sample.

IF YOU AIM TO HANDLE ANY SAMPLE AS IF IT WERE FROM A HIV INFECTED PATEINT THEN THAT IS GOOD CLINICAL PRACTICE (THOUGH YOU DO NOT NEED TO PUT EVERY SAMPLE IN A SPECIAL 'DANGER HIHG RISK BAG).

Medicbyte

Medicbyte

PLAB procedure two

Urethral Catheterisation

When must you think about catherisation?

Urinary retention
In some cases of urinary incontinence
Monitoring fluid balance in certain situations e.g. Post operatively in some cases/ ICU
In children undergoing MCUG procedures

Equipment Required

Kidney dish (for catching urine)
Cleaning fluid (saline) and swabs
Sterile Gloves
(Some doctor's don on two sets of gloves- after leaning the penis they remove the outer set)
Catheter and Catheter bag
Lignocaine Gel
Saline and 10 ml syringe

(1) Prepare the patient

'I need to put this catheter into your bladder and need you to be relaxed so that it is easier to do'

(2) Position the patient supine on a bed.

(3) Choose a relevant catheter. It is best to check that the balloon is working so you may need another set of gloves or you can check it before you put it in.

A general rule is the smallest catheter should be used that provides an adequate urinary channel for the flow of urine to the outside. Generally silicone catheters can be used long term and rubber catheters for short-term catherisation.

(4) Get the instruments. Will need a sterile field and a small pot containing cleaning fluid. Prepare the patient, clean the area and apply lignocaine jelly (0.5%) to the urethra (warn the patient that it may sting) and then wait for 5 minutes.

Remember to do the cleaning with your left hand and all the clean objects are to be handled by your right hand.

(5) Pull the penis upwards so that the urethra is straight and pass the catheter without holding onto the catheter (a forceps may be required). You will come to a point where you will feel pressure, after this there is a give and urine may flow out. Take catheter down to the hilt if you can.

(6) Inflate up the balloon with a syringe (read the label to see how much saline should be pushed into the balloon with 10ml of saline. The balloon mechanism anchors the catheter and stops it from falling out.

(7) Connect the catheter to a closed drainage bag.

Medicbyte

When urine does not flow...

Ask yourself

Have you got the diagnosis of urinary retention correct, could this be anuria due to hepato-renal syndrome, for example.

UK HOSPITALS

In UK hospitals, traditionally, females are catheterised by female nursing/medical staff.

Medicbyte

PLAB procedure three

Skin Suturing

This is an essential skill for all doctors, particularly surgeons- who probably do not need to read this page!! When managing a wound the basic principles are very important. Questions to ask are…

Is the wound clean?
As there are chances of contamination?
Where is the wound and will it heal there?
Does the wound need to be dealt by a plastic surgeon?
Is there any chance that glass may be present here?
Has bleeding been stopped adequately?
Will the patient tolerate local anaesthesia/general anaesthesia?

Certain wounds are best dealt by experts, i.e. plastic surgeons.

For example if an injury has occurred in an area that can have cosmetic consequences e.g. young lady. Children don't like stitches and if the injury is major or in a difficult area they may need to be anaesthetised for the procedure. It may be possible to get by without suturing if cuts are small by using steri-strips or by using special glue to oppose the edges.

Sometimes suturing can be very challenging, e.g. in a drunk individual on a Friday night in the Accident and emergency department.

Suturing in the PLAB examination.

I made sure that I knew exactly what I was doing. I talked through all the steps.

I made sure to remember that the 'make believe skin' was a part of a real patient. So I made comments on ensuring that the patients Airway and Breathing and Circulation were all fine. Then I said I would reassure the patient by informing the patient about what I was doing and the fact that he/she would not feel pain because of the local anaesthetic I was using. I did this all quickly.

The examiner watched me doing the suturing and seemed to be very keen to see how I handled the sharps. I carefully handled the sharps with the suturing equipment and put them into the sharps bin after I had finished them.

Medicbyte

For suturing

(1) Prepare the patient- introduce yourself.

Say to the examiner:-

'I assume that the Airway, Breathing and Circulation have all been assessed and are fine'. I would take a history and examination to look into the mechanism of injury. Further information may be useful as there may be foreign body contamination or an infection risk'

Say to the examiner:-

I will now inform the patient what I am going to do.

'You need a number of stitches to the cut. It is important that you are still for the procedure'

(2) Prepare the instruments

(3) Prepare Yourself- clean and dry hands. WEAR GLOVES. Is the patient cooperative, if not then you will need help, call a nurse.

(3) Clean the wound

(4) Anaesthetise the area (ensure patient has no allergies)

If the patient is not going to receive a general anaesthesia then you will have to apply a local anaesthetic. Usually a mixture containing lignocaine and adrenaline is used as this helps local haemostasis. However if the area is to an end artery supply then the adrenaline mixture cannot be used.

'I am just going to numb your skin with this local anaesthetic, it might sting for a few seconds and then everything will go numb'

The local should be drawn up in a 2ml syringe and applied via a green needle to the area requiring stitching. As you apply the local always remember to suck back on the plunger of the syringe to ensure you are not injecting directly into a blood vessel.

(6)   Prepare the wound

Ensure there are no particles or dirt within the wound.

DON'T USE ADRENALINE CONTAINING LOCAL ANAESTHETICS AROUND THE earlobes, fingers, toes, nasal tip, penis tip because of the HIGH RISK OF ISCHAEMIC NECROSIS

(7)   Oppose the edges to see whether the opposition of the edges will be possible.

TOP TIP

REMEMBER TO WEAR GLOVES. The GMC wish to ensure that you are safe to practice in the UK and at the same time you protect yourself from practices that could be dangerous to you.

Medicbyte

PLAB procedure four

Arterial Blood Gases

This is required to assess the adequacy of breathing and the circulation.

Possible Sites
Radial/Femoral

You will need: Heparinised syringe with a green or blue needle
Alcohol Swab
Cotton wool
Lignocaine as a local anaesthetic (in a 2ml syringe and an 25G needle)
or ametop cream

If there is time and the patient is fully conscious then it is kinder to pre anaesthetise the area; which in the radial approach could be undertaken by anaesthetic cream. The femoral approach is more difficult to anaesthetise.

Radial
Assume comfortable position for the patient and yourself- reassure the patient
Have the patients hand extended with a roll under the wrist; have the area in a flat posture
Perform the Allen test (If patients fails Allen test try other hand)
DO NOT PERFORM PROCEDURE IF ALLEND TEST FAILED
Palpate the artery
Clean area with alcohol swab
Apply lignocaine bleb – remembering to check for inadvertent vascular puncture by the lignocaine (just suck back before you inject the lignocaine- if you see blood you have hit a vessel)
In between your fingers pass the needle vertically until you hit the artery (45-90 degree angles are used for puncture- use what best suits you)
When you hit the artery the syringe will self-fill (take 1-3ml)
With draw the needle and place pressure on the puncture site for 2-3 minutes
Take care when taking the needle off the syringe, get rid of air bubbles and put a cap on the syringe
Label the syringe & take the blood for analysis; if you have to send the blood to another part of the building then place the sample in ICE; label the bag too.

Femoral
Locate the artery with two fingers of your left hand (if you are right handed and vice versa if you are left handed) and fix the artery

Pass the needle vertically between your fingers and as you do so place withdrawal pressure on your syringe until you hit the artery and the syringe will self-fill

Notes
The radial approach is easier to get to, but if there have been previous attempts or in the case of obesity there it may be difficult to palpate the radial artery.

In some hospitals special pre-heparinised syringes are available; if not then heparinise your own syringe with 100 Units of heparin.

Take care in clinical states where there is a bleeding tendency; always say to the examiner. *'I will establish rapport with the patient and also ask pertinent questions looking for contraindications to the procedure- such as a bleeding tendency or medications like Warfarin'.*

Medicbyte

Medicbyte

PLAB procedure five

Blood Pressure Measurement

This may seem like a straightforward task, but due to undue confidence some doctors do this badly! The aim in stations like these, is to score highly so that the difficult stations are not as important in the final scheme of things.

You will need: Choose a BP cuff and sphygmomanometer

The size of the BP cuff should be such that it covers 2/3 of the upper limb when folded.

Method:

Introduce yourself to the patient (have him/her sitting) and sit beside him
Wrap the cuff round the upper arm (always choose the same arm in
                            all your patients for the sake of consistency)
Attach to the sphygmomanometer and have the arm at the level of the heart
Zero the cuff pressure and then inflate whilst palpating the radial pulse on the same side
When the pusle is not felt pump the cuff to at least 25-30 mmHg above the systolic pressure (which you can feel by palpating the radial artery)
Then place the stethoscope in the brachial area auscultating to listen for Kroktov sounds

On deflation	**First sound**	First Korotkof sound	Systolic Pressure
	When you hear the next sound disappear	Korotkof Vth sound	Diastolic Pressure

Finish by saying

'I would also like to measure the blood pressure with the patient standing to look for postural hypotension'

The magic number is a greater than 20-mmHg systolic pressure fall on standing for greater than two minutes implies postural hypotension

Medicbyte

Medicbyte

An Important Tip for Candidates- Stay Sharp!!

When undertaking the skills stations involving Sharps you should be very careful with what you do with sharps.

The examiner is takes great attention to

1. How you handle the sharp.
2. What you when you finish with the sharp.
3. That you know there is a sharps injury policy in case of a sharps injury.
4. That you carry sharps to the sharps bin safely; preferably in a paper tray.
5. That you ensure the sharps bin is not overfull.

Remember the examiner is watching!!

Medicbyte

Medicbyte

Emergency Managment
A B C....Z

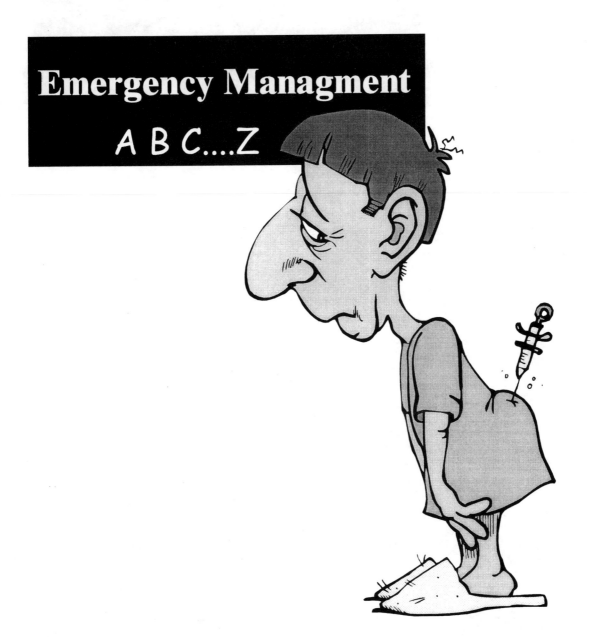

Medicbyte

Medicbyte

Emergency Management

As a doctor working a busy UK hospital you will be required to be competent in basic skills in cardio pulmonary resuscitation. These include airway, breathing and circulatory management.

Scenarios for the testing of your emergency management skills will include

- CPR (adult or child)
- Acute severe asthma
- Primary Survey
- Secondary Survey
- Counsel a mother about a petechial rash over the phone
- Diabetic Ketoacidosis management

The best way to practice these emergency management scenarios is with a group of doctors. There are courses available for the PLAB 2. Ensure that any course you attend has dummies available for CPR practice.

The Medicbyte course provides all the necessary training for the PLAB 2.

TOP TIP
If you are asked to role-play a scenario where you have to describe a sick patient try to present it in a logical coherent manner. A good approach is to start with the Airway then comment on breathing, then circulation and finally the neurology. Say 'starting with the Airway the patient is......'

Medicbyte

Medicbyte

Basic Life Support

Basic life support is the life support offered immediately at a cardiac arrest, advanced life support is for support offered by experts with further equipment to hand.

For the PLAB examination you must be able to demonstrate the following

- Have a safe approach to CPR for yourself and the patient
- Have an ordered approach A B C
- Know when to call for help
- Be able to demonstrate Airway opening techniques
- Be able to demonstrate Breathing techniques which do not under-inflate or over-inflate the lung
- Be able to demonstrate safe external cardiac massage at the correct site and the correct

This section gives a brief summary of CPR for the PLAB examination.

Shout For Help- Say *'Someone Call the Crash Team'*

Make sure you and the patient are safe
Ask the examiner: 'I would ensure that the area is SAFE?'
For example you should not be trying CPR in a patient whom has been electrocuted without turning off the electricity

Check For Response Ask the mannequin: 'Are you all right?'
Check For Breathing, Assess Circulation, start CPR

Airway
Attempt airway opening manoeuvres
Head tilt and Chin Lift

Breathing
Check Adequacy of breathing (for 10 seconds)
Place your ear over the patients mouth so that you can feel a breathe whilst looking at the patients chest for chest movement. If there is a visible obstruction and you think it can be easily removed, then do so. In children never try to remove obstructions.

Give Two Rescue Breathes
Using mouth to mouth ventilation

Circulation
Check Circulation (Carotid Pulse) for 10 seconds

If inadequate circulation then start cardiac compressions

Give 15 compressions with every 2 breathes

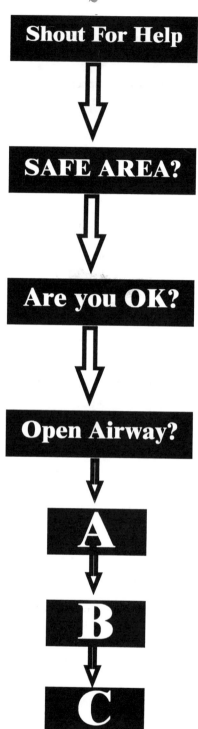

Medicbyte

Shout For Help

SAFE AREA?

Are you OK?

Open Airway?

A

B

C

BLS Medicbyte

Medicbyte

Occasionally you may be required to demonstrate CPR in a child. Below are brief guidelines on differences in the different age groups (one rescuer assumed).

	Infant	**Small Child**	**Large Child/Adult**
A- Neck positioning	Neutral	Sniffing the morning air	Sniffing the morning air
B Initial rescue breathes	Up to 5 Stop when you have given 2 good breathes	5 Up to 5 Stop when you have given 2 good breathes	Up to 5 Stop when you have given 2 good breathes
CPR ratio	5:1	5:1	15:2

Advanced Life Support

It is important that you start basic life support until the rest of the crash team arrive. You should therefore be in a position where you can provide a breathe and give cardiac massage easily.

- Give 100% Oxygen as soon as possible
- Intubate as soon as practical, but giving ventilation via an anaesthetic bag will suffice.

One of the following conditions may be diagnosed

VF or Pulseless VT

Asystole

Pulseless electrical activity

See overleaf for treatment algorithms for each...

Medicbyte

VF or Pulseless VT

Precordial thump
DC shock 200J
DC shock 360J

To undertake the following for as long as defibrillation is indicated

Adrenaline 1mg i.v.
10 CPR or 5:1

DC shock 360J
DC shock 360J
DC shock 360J

Asystole

Precordial thump
Intubate, iv access and 1mg adrenaline iv

10 CPR sequences of 5:1
Atropine 3mg iv once
If no response after three cycles think about giving high dose adrenaline

Causes of Pulseless electrical activity

- *Hypokalaemia*
- *Hypovolaemia*
- *Hypothermia*
- *PE*
- *Pneumothorax*
- *Cardiac Tamponade*
- *Drug overdose*

Note
Pulseless electrical activity used to be called electro-mechanical dissociation. Always check that the monitoring is fixed properely to the patient before starting CPR as sometimes this is the casuse of a chaotic wave form on the monitor.

Medicbyte

Trauma Life Support

A comprehensive review of trauma care is beyond the scope of the PLAB however there are certain clinical scenarios you should be able to perform. These are listed below:-

- Perform a Glasgow Coma Score assessment
- Perform a Primary Survey
- Perform a Secondary Survey
- Know what a trauma X-ray series is. (Simply this is a Cervical-spine/ CXR and Pelvis X-ray)

Glasgow Coma Score

Eye Opening

Spontaneous	4
To Voice	3
To Pain	2
No Response	1

Best Motor Response

Obeys verbal command	6	
Localizes to pain	5	
Withdraws to pain	4	
Abnormal flexion to pain	3	(decorticate)
Abnormal extension to pain	2	(decerebrate)
No response to pain	1	

Best Verbal response

Converses and orientated	5
Converses but disorientated	4
Inappropriate Words	3
Incomprehensible words	2
No response to pain	1

Medicbyte

Primary Survey

This is the initial survey that is required when a casualty arrives through the door. The aim is to assess quickly and perform life saving acts such as airway management; ventilation with bag and mask and external cardiac massage. An assessment of the neurological system must be made quickly (D for disability).

A
B
C
D

Secondary Survey

The secondary survey is put into action when the casualty has been stabilized and then you need to think about what could cause further problems (e.g. an impending pneumothroax or a femoral fracture with torrential bleed).

The secondary survey involves a focused medical history, clinical examination and investigations.

Medicbyte

On the Day and After

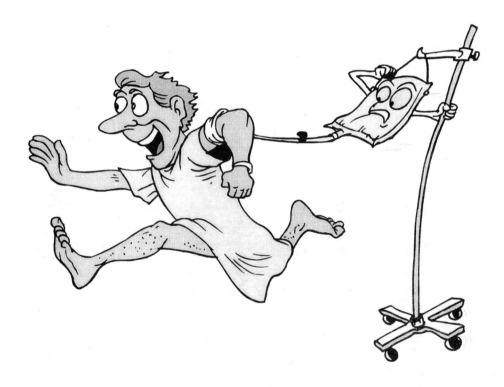

Medicbyte

Medicbyte

On the day

This may be a stressful day, but remember there is a high pass rate....you have got this far and there is no reason why you can't pass. You have nothing to lose with this positive attitude.

So you've trained for it and the day has arrived. This chapter will give you tips on how to get through the day unscathed.

Where is the examination?

The PLAB 2 examination can only be taken in the United Kingdom and there are a number of centres. You should be given enough information by the GMC about this prior to the examination.

Where should you stay?

When should you arrive?

How long does the exam last?

There are 14 stations of 5 minutes each. You have a minute before each station to read the instructions concerning your next station. In total though, from start to finish the duration is one hour and thirty-six minutes.

Remember to bring your proof of identity..

Please see the GMC examination regulations for this.

Medicbyte

If you fail

You have a total of four goes for the PLAB 2. If you fail then you will have to undertake the IELTS examination and the PLAB 1 again. So it is best to focus on passing.

Like anything that you do in life, which involves patients, you must demand excellence in yourself so that you can give the best care to your patients. If you only just failed then this is encouraging. However what ever your mark you should be using this 'failure' as a wake-up call.

Consequently if you fail you must ask yourself what are your failings?

Why is it that separate doctors at each station have expected more from you.

Why didn't you give enough to your patient?

Was it a problem with knowledge?

Were you really nervous on the day? How can you overcome this the next time?

A self-analysis is called for at this point. This is best done by going over, with experienced colleagues, the stations that you came across in the examination. If you have no-one to talk to then you can book an online-session with one of the Medicbyte teachers email **passplab@medicbyte.com**

Medicbyte

Case Study: An example of a student's problems in the examination.

I got a distressed phone call from a doctor (who had not taken our PLAB 2 course) Her failings are detailed below:-

1. Really nervous on the day.

I reassured her that the next time she will do better because she has already been through the experience. Repletion is the mother of skill.

2. Her approach to clinical management issues seemed haphazard.

I told her that when dealing with sick patients, no matter what the illness, she should have a ABCD approach.

A   Airway

B   Breathing

C   Circulation

D   Disability

Also when discussing the problems with colleagues she should think about summarizing the problem in a ABCD like-manner purely because this is the way doctors are taught in the UK.

3.   She ran out of time during the examination of one of the systems.

Repetition is the mother of skill. Practicing on a teddy bear; talking to Harry the cat are examples of how doctors have prepared for postgraduate examinations.

You do not have time in the examination to dilly-dally about what's next in clinical examination. The procedures of clinical examination should have been embedded into you in at spinal root level!!

Medicbyte

Medicbyte

Working as a Doctor in the UK
Passed the PLAB 2; now what?

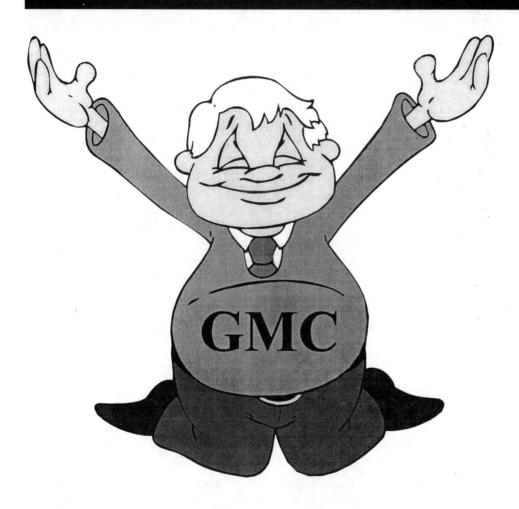

Medicbyte

Never forget the hours you spent struggling over the PLAB, other obstacles will come your way but these too you can overcome if you have the same conviction in yourself.

Medicbyte PLAB Services

Medicbyte

Medicbyte

Unfortunately, passing the PLAB does not guarantee you work as a doctor. There are still a number of hurdles to overcome, but at least you have passed a UK based examination system.

Below are a list of important considerations:

(1) Getting a SHO job

This can be a difficult task, you will first have to have UK referees and then you must write to as many hospitals in the speciality you are interested.

This can itself be a soul-destroying exercise but keep at it!

(2) Medico-legal indemnity

Once you start work you will have to join a union that will protect your interest should there be ever any reason for anyone to take you to court. **This is highly recommended**

(3) British Medical Association

Joining the BMA can also give you a number of important benefits.

(4) Adjusting to a different way of working

There will be different demands from you from all areas including nursing staff and patients. It is important o be courteous at all times.

Remember there will be things about your previous medical system, if you have previously worked abroad, that will show that you have indeed skills to offer to the medical system.

Please visit the Medicbyte website where there are a number of facilities for doctors looking for a placement in the United Kingdom.

The National Health Service also arranges induction courses for doctors who have passed PLAB and will be working in UK hospitals- to find out about these contact the postgraduate medical deans office in your local area.

Practicing medicine in the United Kingdom my, at first, seem a daunting task. However the PLAB 1 and 2 examinations have been designed so that you can acclimatize to the new environment without too many problems.

FOR MORE TIPS ON FINDING WORK AFTER PLAB SEE Dr Asima's Book

Medicbyte

Medicbyte

Appendix

Using the CDROM: The exclusive PLAB area of the website

The CDROM provides you with an extra dimension to connect to the medicbyte website where you will find further helpful advice for the purposes of personal study.

To use the CDROM you should connect to the Internet and then clicking on the relevant links will take you into the exclusive PLAB area of the website.

You must have speaker and audio capability on your computer to fully utilize the material provided.

PLAB 2 Course

Medicbyte holds courses for the PLAB in the United Kingdom and at centres abroad. Medicbyte teachers are experienced teachers for the PLAB examination.

The PLAB 2 course provides candidates with invaluable experience and feedback to pass the final examination.

More details on course venues etc are provided on the website at www.medicbyte.com

PLAB 2 Video CDROMS

CDROMS illustrating clinical examinations are available from Medicbyte. These videos demonstrate the practical skills you require to pass the PLAB 2.

Included are the following sections: -

Clinical Examination: Respiratory System
Clinical Examination: Gastrointestinal System
Clinical Examination: Cardiovascular System
Clinical Examination: Neurological System
Practical Procedures
Basic Life Support
Joint examination for the PLAB
Communication for the PLAB examination

Please see the website for details at www.medicbyte.com

Medicbyte

Medicbyte PLAB 2 Course: the final approach

Experienced UK clinicians supervise the Medicbyte PLAB 2 courses.

The latest manikins based interactive media are used at the centres.

(1) Tutor Based Intensive PLAB II weekend Course

Day 1

0930-0945 Introduction

1000-1115 Resuscitation

1130-1200 Practical Procedures 1

1200-1300 Surgery

1245-1400 Lunch

1400-1515 Clinical Skills 1

1600-1700 Practical Procedures 2 and Scenarios

Day 2

0930-0945 Resuscitation 2

1000-1030 Practical Procedures 3

1030-1130 General Medicine 1

1130-1245 General Medicine 2

1245-1401 Lunch

1400-1515 O&G and VE

1600-1700 Practical Procedures 2

Medicbyte

Day 1

Resuscitation 1	Basic Life support (practice with manikin)
	BP measurement
	Paediatric Resuscitation

Practical Procedures 1   IV access and venepuncture

Surgery	Scenario
	Practice PR exam with manikins
	Testicular exam
	Urinary catheter placement

Clinical Skills 1   History; exam and scenarios

Practical Procedures 2   Stitching + miscellaneous

Day 2

Resuscitation 2   Advanced Life support

Practical procedures 3   Asthma, inhalers, peak flow

General Medicine 1   Respiratory and GI and CVS

General Medicine 2   Neurology

O&G and VE	Breast examination
	Scenarios
	Vaginal examination

Please see www.medicbyte.com for the latest program details or Contact Medicbyte UK.

Medicbyte

Medicbyte

Career Services

- Medicbyte Provides books/online courses/DVD's and VHS videos for PLAB training
- Courses are also available at the Medicbyte Centre
- Locum Services and Attachment services
- Accommodation

Contact us today!

Why not take a read of the Career Guide by Medicbyte

HOW TO GET A JOB AFTER PLAB

After passing the PLAB examination the next task is to find work in the UK. How to go about it, wher to look, how to prepare for interview and how to fill in the forms- everything is discussed by Dr Asima Rashid GP Registrar (Bedfordshire). Buy this book and save time and increase your chances of work in any field.

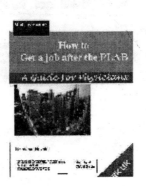

Provides important tips that will save you time.

Medicbyte

Medicbyte PLAB (I) EMQ Course Theory and Practice

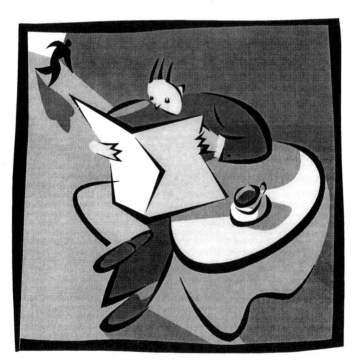

Course by Medicbyte
www.medicbyte.com

Course Dates: **At regular intervals before each examination**

Medicbyte

Contact: plab@medicbyte.com
www.medicbyte.com

Medicbyte Books/Videos/DVD's/Courses

PLAB 1 Book 1

Medicbyte PLAB books contain up-to-date information for the PLAB. Each book contains questions with answers detailing important PLAB concepts. Written by UK doctors and therefore are ideal for the clinical scenarios for the PLAB examination. Now all Revised for 2004 so that you can be ahead of your competition. You must score better than the mean score for your exam date to pass, Medicbyte books show you how!

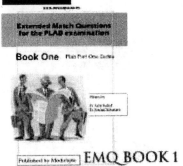

2003 Edition with CDROM!

PLAB 1 Book 2

Builds on Book 1 to cover more important concepts for the PLAB examination.

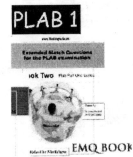

2003 Edition

PLAB 1 Book 3

The final book in the PLAB 1 series completes the series for the PLAB

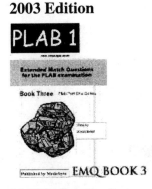

2003 Edition

Medicbyte

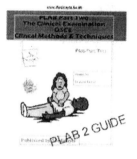

PLAB 1 Online Course
Course Designed on the PLAB 1
Intensive weekend course by Medicbyte

2003 Edition

PLAB 1 Special Discount
Buy all the PLAB 1 books by
Medicbyte!

ALL 3 Books

PLAB 2 Book
Clinical book for the PLAB 2 with Hot
topics and tips for every aspect of the
PLAB

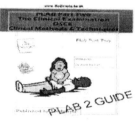

With CDROM

PLAB 1 & 2 Special Discount
Buy all the PLAB 1 & 2 books by
Medicbyte!

ALL 4 Books

PLAB 2 Fast-track Course
Medicbyte PLAB 2 course fast track This
course is designed to give doctors
practice vital for the PLAB 2 The course
is a hands-on session only (a PLAB 2
doctor who has passed the exam
recently will be present to give helpful
tips). PLAB 2 book is also provided.
Contact Medicbyte for dates.

With CDROM

PLAB 2 Videos (Full Set of 4 VHS Videos) + PLAB 2 Book
Medicbyte PLAB 2 Videos (Procedures &
techniques for the PLAB 2) Blood taking
& cannulation primary and secondary
survey Knee exam Vaginal exam using
the speculum Breast exam Urinary
Catherisation (Clinical Examination)
Introduction CVS RESPIRATORY
GASTROINTESTINAL RECTAL BP CNS (I
AND II) HIP & KNEE EXAMINATION
Price For Full Set

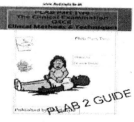

Medicbyte

4 VHS Videos

<u>ORDER FORMS</u>

Medicbyte

Medicbyte Book order form
PLAB Books 1/2/3 Discount pack (online orders only)
PLAB Book 1 (with CDROM)
PLAB Book 2
PLAB Book 3
PLAB 1 online Course
PLAB 2 Book
PLAB 1 & 2 Discount Pack (online orders only)
PLAB 2 Videos (+free PLAB 2book)
MRCPCH Book
How to get a job after PLAB
How to work in the USA
Clinical Skills Examination USA Licensure for doctors
Prices are subject to change without notice.

Card Number: | | | | | | | | | | | | | | | | | **Expiry Date:** | | |

Issue No.: | | | **Valid From:** | | | **Security Card No. :** | | |

(3 digit number found on/below the signature strip)

Name (as shown on card):

PLEASE PRINT NAME

Registered Address of Card Holder:

PLEASE PRINT ADDRESS

Signature of cardholder:

Please check the website for details of the extensive overseas centres.